Comprehensive Disability Management

Commissioning Editor: Susan Young
Development Editor: Catherine Jackson
Project Manager: Caroline Horton
Designer: George Ajayi
Illustration Manager: Bruce Hogarth

Comprehensive Disability Management

Henry G. Harder EdD, RPsych

Associate Professor, Chair, Disability Management and Psychology Programs, University of Northern British Columbia, Prince George, British Columbia, Canada

Liz R. Scott PhD, MEng, MBA, MSc, BSc, RN, COHN-C, COHN-S, CRSP, CDMP

Principal, Organizational Solutions, Burlington, Ontario, and part-time lecturer at Ryerson University Toronto, and McGill University, Montreal, Canada

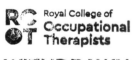

Royal College of **Occupational Therapists**

WITHDRAWN

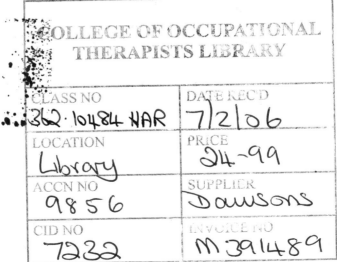
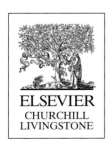

ELSEVIER
CHURCHILL
LIVINGSTONE

EDINBURGH LONDON NEW YORK OXFORD PHILADELPHIA ST LOUIS SYDNEY TORONTO 2005

ELSEVIER
CHURCHILL
LIVINGSTONE

First published 2005

ISBN 0 443 10113 2

British Library Cataloguing in Publication Data
A catalogue record for this book is available from the British Library

Library of Congress Cataloging in Publication Data
A catalog record for this book is available from the Library of Congress

Notice
Neither the Publisher nor the Authors assume any responsibility for any loss or injury and/or damage to persons or property arising out of or related to any use of the material contained in this book. It is the responsibility of the treating practitioner, relying on independent expertise and knowledge of the patient, to determine the best treatment and method of application for the patient.

The Publisher

Working together to grow
libraries in developing countries

www.elsevier.com | www.bookaid.org | www.sabre.org

ELSEVIER BOOK AID International Sabre Foundation

ELSEVIER your source for books, journals and multimedia in the health sciences
www.elsevierhealth.com

Printed in China

We dedicate this book to:

Our families for their unebbing support and tolerance, and their knowledge that chasing dreams is a constant activity in our lives;

Our friends for their significant and energizing contributions;

All disability management professionals for their ongoing quest for fairness and equity;

Each other for our hard work and our ability to work together and become friends.

Contents

Introduction

Disability management (DM) is a new and emerging discipline. The value in DM has been recognized throughout the industrialized world and the practice of DM has been eagerly embraced by employers and a vast array of professionals. DM is now practised by occupational therapists, kinesiologists, nurses, insurance specialists, psychologists, rehabilitation professionals and those with no particular training. As professionals, DM practitioners have a significant impact on the financial and human costs of disability. Most major corporations have the need for a DM programme and therefore require individuals with the skills, capability and knowledge to perform these functions. The financial cost of disability in corporations is one of the key target areas that requires attention. The human costs of disability are also quite dramatic and efforts need to be geared towards reducing the impact of disabilities on individuals. Given the importance of this task it is remarkable that more resources and education have not been provided. That has begun to change.

It has been recognized that specific training in DM is necessary if the new emerging profession is going to sustain its growth and continue to develop and mature into a fully recognized profession. Consequently, there are now courses in DM, at various levels of academia, being offered in Europe, Canada, the USA and Australia. This explosion in education, and a burgeoning of DM as a career choice, has revealed a lack of adequate resources for teaching purposes. This book is aimed at that lack and will make a valuable contribution to students, academics and DM practitioners.

We begin the book with an overview of the history of DM. We then introduce a systems-based theoretical model in this developing profession and provide practical examples of how to implement and manage an effective DM programme. We go on to cover the entire spectrum of DM including role definitions, discussions on key components, communication, claim initiation, claims management, return to work, rehabilitation, data analysis, workplace culture, quality assurance and full programme evaluation. The book is comprehensive, encompassing the entire spectrum of disability from prevention to return to work, as we believe that successful DM is Comprehensive Disability Management.

INTENDED AUDIENCE

This book is intended for university level (credit and non-credit) courses in Disability Management and as a resource for DM practitioners.

This book will also be of interest to insurance companies, workers' compensation boards, third-party administrators and consultants in DM.

OVERVIEW

Chapter 1 will help the reader understand the evolution of DM. It contains a review of how individuals with disabilities have been treated in the past, including the attitudes of society that allowed such treatment. Further, it reviews the progress made to date in the field of DM.

Chapter 2 outlines the critical components of DM. We provide all of the essential components necessary for successful DM, from prevention to return to work emphasizing the need for data analysis and programme evaluation.

Chapter 3 contains the presentation of a systems-based conceptual model of DM. The workplace and individual lives are extremely complicated in today's society. This model recognizes and places great importance on the DM practitioners being familiar with, and working effectively within, an environment filled with these many complexities. We stress the importance of dealing with the entire person, including their entire personal network.

Chapter 4 outlines how DM functions within an organization. In order to place this within an appropriate context we review the basic operations of an organization, including how an organization plans, sets goal and objectives, and how these are evaluated.

Chapter 5 stresses the importance of prevention, health and safety. The key components of health, safety and health promotion are discussed as is the importance of having a corporate culture that embraces and supports such initiatives. The importance of prevention and DM being linked is also discussed.

Chapter 6 looks at the importance of programme development that is performed well. We stress the importance of developing policies and procedures and the skills and knowledge necessary to do so. The importance of defining the roles within a programme and who will fill the roles is also stressed.

Chapter 7 is a key chapter focusing on the importance of early intervention. The factors that underlie the importance of early intervention are clearly identified and discussed in detail. Particular attention is paid to the critical importance of psychosocial factors. Different models of rehabilitation are also discussed.

Chapter 8 discusses the critical nature of accurate and timely claim initiation. The importance of accurate form completion and the consequences of sloppy work are discussed. We look at the differences between occupational and non-occupational claims initiation, processing and management.

Chapter 9 discusses and defines the different nuances to case and claim management. We explore the case and claim management process including the importance of effective and accurate case monitoring. Further, we outline the potential impact of case management when it is well done.

Chapter 10 focuses on probably the most active components of DM: return to work (i.e. RTW). We discuss the different complexities inherent in facilitation RTW and the key factor of recognizing when to bridge the gap between recovery and RTW.

Chapter 11 brings us up to date in the area of rehabilitation. This chapter outlines the development of medical and vocational rehabilitation and discusses their strengths and weaknesses. It also deals with the importance of providing rehabilitation for psychosocial issues.

Chapter 12 examines the very interesting area of the duty to accommodate. Key legislation on jurisprudence in support of the duty to accommodate is presented. The obligations of all parties under this duty are presented, and the implications of non-compliance are discussed.

Chapter 13 presents the importance of programme evaluation. Effective programme design requires needs evaluation, process evaluation and summative evaluation in order to provide appropriate services and to show the efficacy of the programme. We present examples of how this can be done and suggest who best to do it. Key tips on report writing and presentation are reviewed; the key nature of evaluation is stressed.

Chapter 14 focuses on the very important and often under-stressed area of communication. Everyone assumes they can communicate yet few people do it very well. Communication is arguably the most important aspect of DM. In this chapter we examine the importance of interactions between all the participants in the DM process and suggest a model for effective communication.

Chapter 15 delves into the area of ethics. In this chapter we discuss the origins of ethics, how we decided on what constitutes ethical behaviour and the development of professional codes of ethics. Specific ethics issues such as confidentiality and informed consent are also discussed. Two existing codes of ethics are presented.

Chapter 16 focuses on future trends in DM. We asked eight professionals – from industry, consulting, organized labour and academia, who are well versed in DM and who are located around the world – to comment on what they see the future holding for DM. Their very insightful thoughts are presented and are worthy of profound reflection.

SUMMARY

The authors hope that you, the reader, will not only find this book of interest but that it will become a valued resource that you will use in your practice of DM regardless of what area you function in. It is our wish that this book fill the gap and provide you with the tools required to function successfully in the field of comprehensive disability management.

Chapter **1**

History and evolution of disability management

LEARNING OBJECTIVES

- Understand the evolution of the disability management movement
- Review the treatment of individuals with disabilities
- Review the evolution of attitudes and treatment of disability in society
- Review the continual progression of disability management

INTRODUCTION

In many ways 1980 was the seminal year for disability management (DM). In that year the World Rehabilitation Fund held the International Exchange of Information in Rehabilitation. Many factors led to the organizers deciding there was a need for such a gathering including the Rehabilitation Act of 1973 (and its Amendments in 1978) and efforts by the World Health Organization (WHO) in 1973 and 1985 to draw attention to the issues of people with disabilities.

At that gathering Jarvikoski and Lahelma (1980), speaking of their pioneering work in early rehabilitation, defined DM as a coordinated activity which:

- is directed toward an individual with a chronic or permanent functional limitation or disability, or an individual with symptoms indicating a risk of chronic functional limitations or disability
- is intended to restore an individual's working or functional capacity, or prevent its lowering
- includes measures aimed at developing an individual's own resources or removing obstacles imposed by the environment.

By providing this definition with its focus on activity they set the stage for others such as policy-makers, business and labour leaders, healthcare professionals and academics to begin the process of putting these notions into practice and DM was born.

But why was this type of activity necessary? What were the driving forces behind this activity? In order to answer these questions we must understand the history of disability and through such understanding begin to comprehend the experience of those living with disability.

HISTORICAL CONTEXT

There is anthropological evidence showing that people with disabilities have been included in society since prehistoric times. Hahn and Kleinman (1983) give as an example the case of bodily remains which clearly showed deformity but whose burial site indicated that the community had held this person in high esteem.

With industrialization came a new attitude toward disability. Whereas people with disabilities had been primarily cared for by family members in the home up to this time, the new demands of the industrial age required people to leave their homes and pursue employment in factories, which meant that no one was left at home to take care of a relative with a disability. Also, in pre-industrialized society a person with a disability may have been able to contribute to the family's business such as farming or baking. The new industrialized jobs, however, did not make accommodations for people with disabilities. These factors meant that such individuals lost their places in society, and the corresponding increase in the difficulty of taking care of family members with disabilities led society to conclude that the solution was the institutionalization of people with disabilities.

Initial efforts at institutionalization were modelled on Elizabethan poor laws. These laws provided for the care of individuals who could no longer be cared for by their families and were now considered an unproductive drain on society. Thus people with disabilities became part of society's underclass, considered to be defective, unhealthy, deviant and requiring special care in order to survive (Garland 1995). By the middle of the nineteenth century it had become apparent that these catch-all institutions did not meet the needs of all residents, and special institutions – such as those for the deaf or blind – were created. While the motivation for such action was seen to put people 'suffering' from a disability with those 'suffering' a similar disability the result was that people with disabilities were removed from general society. This movement gathered force with the advent of Social Darwinism, which advanced the notion that people with disabilities were defective and should be removed from view and isolated from society. This idea received further support from the writings of Francis Galton (1901) who is credited with the birth of eugenics. He stated that eugenics should be 'the study of agencies under social control that may improve or impair the racial qualities of future generations, either physically or mentally . . . a science which deals with all influences that improve and develop inborn qualities of race' (Galton 1904: 82). Thus people with disabilities are to be bred out of existence. This thinking culminated in programmes such as forced sterilization or in extreme cases infanticide or euthanasia to keep the disabled from breeding and weakening the race. Eugenics' ultimate manifestation came at the hands of the Nazi regime and the attempted mass extermination of the Jews and others, including those with disabilities, determined not to fit the ideal of the perfect physical and mental human specimen.

Due in large part to such atrocities eugenics was discredited but it has not disappeared completely and some say it is raising its head again under the guise of the new genetics (Otlowski & Williamson 2003). Advances in genetic research and its application in practical situations is altering how we see health. Once, we cured illness after it was detected. Now we are proposing to eradicate illness by gene therapy or genetic manipulation. Couples are being counselled to abort a disabled fetus or discouraged from having children if either or both of them are genetically predisposed to having a child with a disability. Society is avoiding the label of eugenics for this 'advance' by viewing this as a personal rather than a societal choice. It is argued that no one is being coerced into such action and therefore the new genetics is not eugenics (Richards 2004). How far are we from that application of eugenics when insurance companies refuse to provide healthcare insurance to individuals who may be genetically predisposed to an illness or disability, or an employer who refuses to employ someone who is genetically predisposed to physical or mental illness? Great controversy has raged over the prospect of this practice to the extent that the Netherlands placed a moratorium on genetic testing for insurance purposes in order to deal with public fears (Otlowski & Williamson 2003).

Disability management has primarily been concerned with return to work post-injury or -illness. This narrow focus is expanding to include people with disabilities who have never entered the workforce and disability issues in general. Nevertheless, its strength and uniqueness derive from its activity in the workplace and its emphasis in finding solutions to disability-related issues in the workplace. So why should DM be concerned with the above? After all, most of its clients began life without a disability. Just as unscrupulous employers embraced eugenics early in the twentieth century to justify attacks on union activists and other 'undesirables', it is just as possible for unscrupulous employers to use genetic screening tools to screen out prospective employees or to deny benefits to someone injured at the job. Does this seem farfetched? Imagine a man who injures his back and undergoes a genetic investigation. It is determined that through his genetic history he was predisposed to have a back injury, therefore the injury is not work-related and therefore not valid for compensation. Or consider the case of someone who is absent from work due to stress, which is diagnosed as depression. Again, genetic testing reveals a genetic predisposition to depression and benefits are denied or if this had happened before employment they may never have become employed.

One factor that may arise out of such conditions is that people may refuse to comply with genetic testing and therefore lose the health benefits for conditions that may genuinely be present. A person once labelled as a genetically deficient may never be employed and may never be able to obtain health insurance. Is it hard to comprehend why a person may hide their disability? In the nineteenth century, people with disabilities were considered to be freaks and deviants best removed from the eyes and conscience of society. In the twentieth century, society tried to embrace disability and make people with disabilities contributing members of society. In the twenty-first century we are moving toward eliminating genetic disability. Given this history is it any wonder why people with disabilities may be reticent to expose their vulnerabilities, especially those who have acquired a disability later in life who may have had some very negative attitudes to disability themselves and why it is still true that such people with disabilities – whether congenital or acquired – are still considered among that section of society that is the most disenfranchised and discriminated against.

THE INFLUENCE OF WAR

One group that stands in minor opposition to the above assertion comprises disabled war veterans. It has been said that war is the best way to create people with disabilities. Initially these were thought only to be physical disabilities but are now widely accepted to be psychological as well. War veterans have often advanced advocacy for specific war veteran issues which have also benefited the general disability community (Kudlick 2003). Certainly, advances in battlefield medicine have meant that more soldiers survive their injuries and eventually return home, some with very visible disabilities. While society has also tried to push these veterans aside and hide them in hospitals or institutions this has proved to be more difficult in recent times given the ease with which general information and, more to the point, specific political messages can be circulated. These veterans, particularly those returning from World War II, caused society to examine what it was doing with those who returned with disabilities and also with those deemed to be termed 'less fortunate'.

SOCIAL WELFARE

We can see, in the post-World War II Western world, a focus on and an expansion of welfare systems to compensate for disability. The experienced horror of the war caused a corresponding desire to express a more humanistic approach to solving problems and a desire to see this approach enshrined in governmental policies. During this time we could see the creation of state-sponsored disability insurance and rehabilitation programmes, which were seen as both humane and cost-effective (Berkowitz & McQuaid 1980). For example, in 1956 the USA created Social Security Disability Insurance and in 1966 Canada introduced Canada Pension Plan Disability Benefits. Both of these plans required permanent disability and for the recipient to be totally unemployable. However, all was not well with these plans. Both plans worked in contradiction to vocational rehabilitation (Rubin et al 1995). In order to qualify for vocational rehabilitation assistance a person had to be ready and able to work. If they took any work their disability benefits were terminated even if they could not maintain that employment. This conundrum caused many people to passively accept their lot rather than try to access the workforce.

THE RIGHTS MOVEMENT

Beginning in the 1960s people with disabilities began advocating for their rights. Media attention was (and continues to be) focused on discrimination in race, gender and sexual orientation, not on disability. In 1962 the world watched as James Meredith was escorted onto the campus of Mississippi State University, thereby becoming the first African-American to set foot on a previously 'Whites-only' campus. This scene was replayed over and over again and wired on news shows around the world.

However, no such attention was focused on Ed Roberts when, that same fall, he became the first person with serious multiple disabilities to be enrolled at the University of California Berkeley (McCarthy 2003). This event is seen by many as the beginning of the disability rights (DR) movement, which culminated in the passing of the Americans with Disabilities Act (ADA) in 1990. The purpose of this act is to grant people with disabilities the same guarantees of equal access that the people of colour had been granted through the Civil Rights Act. The ADA prohibits discrimination in areas such as education, access and employment. It gives those working in the field some leverage to begin effecting change in their respective areas. It should be noted that the impact of the ADA has been felt around the world and that advocates in other parts of the world have used the ADA to create changes in their own country.

While the unfolding decades witnessed a worldwide receptiveness to and awareness of the issues facing people with disabilities brought about largely by the work of individual activists and disability rights groups, there was also a growing concern of the magnitude of the problem. As more and more systems were put into place to deal with disability issues, questions about the efficacy of these systems were raised. These questions struck at the core of the disability movement and were in relation to issues such as:

- the definition of what constitutes a disability
- the integrity of the compensation systems that base eligibility on the withdrawal from the workforce
- the adequacy and orientation of various rehabilitation systems
- the limitation of the medical model to deal effectively with issues of disability
- where and how prevention measures should be focused to best facilitate the social integration of people with disabilities.

The WHO Expert Committee, in their 1976 and 1981 reports, reviewed the definitions of terms and concepts related to disability. Given the many definitions of terms used throughout the world the committee suggested that the definitions of three terms be standardized around the following definitions:

- Impairment – any loss or abnormality of psychological, physiological or anatomical structure or function.
- Disability – any restriction or lack of ability to perform an activity in the manner or within the range considered normal.

■ Handicap – a disadvantage for a given individual, resulting from an impairment or disability, which limits or prevents the fulfilment of a role that is normal for the individual.

While it was a noble intention to coalesce around these definitions, they did not resolve pre-existing inherent difficulties. For example, Blaxter (1975) points out the difficulty in objectively defining a term such as 'disability' when he states 'a given impairment may or may not result in functional disablement'. This is a problem when eligibility for compensation is based on 'loss of faculty' and not loss of function. Nagi (1969) discusses the inequities of early systems that relied on schedules of impairment to determine compensation, presuming that the functional impact of impairment could be neatly standardized. This point, which is just as relevant today, is whether compensation should represent payment for the injury or disease when it was sustained or whether payment should be for loss of future income which has come about because of the injury or illness.

COSTS OF DISABILITY

The 1981 United Nations report concluded that the working capacity of a country can be severely reduced if it does not deal with disability-related issues effectively. They further concluded that effective rehabilitation of those with disabilities can provide an important reserve of workers for an economy but that this strength may only become apparent at the time when an economy experiences a labour shortage. Van Hooser and Rice (1989) built on this point, arguing that it is important to build an employment strategy that includes mechanisms for integrating people with disabilities into the workforce. At the time it was becoming increasingly clear that the traditional solution of requiring people with disabilities to remove themselves from the workforce was not an efficient use of person power given the development of global competition, labour shortages (especially in skilled trades), improved technology and the ever-increasing costs of providing benefits to those not in the workforce. It was becoming clear to employers that it was expedient, as well as morally agreeable, to view all employees, including those with disabilities, as a valuable resource worth retaining.

From an international perspective the report identified a common theme that transfer payments to people with disabilities were not helping the situation. In fact, these payments were rewarding incapacity, paying people to stay away from work rather than assisting them to work. Further, these programmes paid little attention to preventing disability nor did they provide incentives for recovery or re-employment. They stated that removing people with disabilities from the workplace and giving them transfer payments cost society more than it would have done to adapt the labour market to meet the needs of people with disabilities. Around the time that these insights were taking place, organizations such as the Disabled People's International were finding ways to advocate for fundamental rights toward full and equal participation of people with disabilities in the workforce and society in general. This resulted in the beginning of a gradual attitudinal shift in communities, which in turn created policy changes, affirmative action programmes and research directed at identifying and eliminating barriers that prevented full and equal participation in society.

Without exception in the Western developed world the models of insurance and transfer payments depend on the medicalization of disability. Hershenson (2000) points out that this fact alone presents a major challenge. In his discourse on cultural anthropology and disability he describes the medical model as one of diagnosis and cure of pathology. He also refers to Stein (1979) who argues that people with permanent disabilities and chronic illnesses represent a threat to the functions of diagnosis and cure of pathology and are therefore outside its scope. This has, of course, not stopped the medical system from treating people with disabilities in the medical model, which, in turn, has resulted in many non-pathological conditions being made pathological so that they could be treated in the medical model. Anyone involved in the broader rehabilitation field is aware of this Catch-22 situation.

Take, for example, the ubiquitous low back strain. A person sustaining a low back strain enters the medical system for treatment. Initially this is appropriate. If the patient does not recover in the appropriate amount of time the medical model does not know what to do with them. It is not uncommon for the physician or physicians to have exhausted all methods of diagnosis without finding one. As a result, there is no pathology to cure. Nevertheless, attempts at treatment take place, usually pharmacological, most often without success. In some cases surgery occurs despite the fact that there is no diagnosis to identify where the surgery should take place or what it should cut out. Study after study (e.g. Habeck et al 1998, Hogg-Johnson & Cole 2003) have shown that the delays in recovery are associated with psychosocial issues that require psychological treatment. Yet we as a society are so fixated on the medical model that other forms of treatment are rarely provided.

This phenomenon has direct implications for the practice of DM. The medical model seeks to return everyone to 'normal'. Clearly this is not possible for people with permanent disabilities, chronic conditions or illnesses. This desire to normalize must be replaced with an individualized, context-specific orientation that aims to achieve flexibility and the skills necessary to integrate comfortably at a level of interdependence, dependence or independence which is specifically unique to each situation.

The contrast between the rehabilitative model and medical model is not new. Many years ago, Anderson (1975) pointed out the shortcomings of the medical model when it is employed for rehabilitative purposes. While describing rehabilitation as a helping profession that requires the active participation of the client, he stated that, clearly, rehabilitation does not eradicate disease or cure the client. Ideally, rehabilitation works cooperatively with the client to gain insight and explore options for problem-solving. Disability management takes this a step further, emphasizing the need to work with all parties involved, including the physicians, in order to not only help the client fully recover but also to return to a productive life. This is in sharp contrast to the medical model which to this day is still based on the authority of the physician and the passivity, acceptance and dependence of the client/patient.

Along with challenging the medical model the timing of the provision of rehabilitation services was also being challenged. It was suggested that rehabilitation interventions would be of greater benefit if they could be initiated before the employment relationship was severed. This was in contrast to the common practice of requiring the person with the disability to remove him- or herself from the workforce. The World Health Organization (1981) stated that the aim of rehabilitation should be to reduce the impact of disabling and handicapping conditions and identified three levels of action required to bring this about:

1. reducing the occurrence of impairments
2. limiting or reversing disability caused by impairment
3. preventing the transition of disability to handicap.

In order for this to happen traditional rehabilitation, with its emphasis on restoration, would have to shift to a preventative focus. In essence the goal of rehabilitation must shift from restoring function alone to also embracing the need to maintain working capacity and the connectedness with the workplace.

In the USA the beginning of this shift was seen in the Rehabilitation Act of 1973. Under this legislation the competency model of restorative rehabilitation was to replace the vocational model such that the object of rehabilitation was no longer vocational readiness but rather competency in independent daily living. The US government concentrated resources toward those with more severe disabilities and away from those with less severe disabilities and those whose functional abilities were progressively deteriorating. In Canada, the Human Rights Code of 1980 legislated equal treatment for individuals with permanent disabilities. The effect of these and subsequent changes led to the development of a private sector of rehabilitation providers who focused on preventative rehabilitation servicing those who had acquired disabilities through work, ageing or disease. Within this context and when the goal is to prevent the movement to unemployment and resulting dependency on transfer payments, the logical and expedient place to intervene is in the workplace. This direction was supported early on by the research of Jarvikoski and Lahelma (1980), Akabas (1986), Mitchell (2002), Galvin (1986) and Schwartz (1984). Disability management has continued to evolve and has accumulated evidence-based research to support interventions to prevent permanent impairment.

CONCLUSION

These pioneers clearly demonstrated that the interplay between business needs, attitudinal changes and rehabilitation could benefit the person with the disability, the employer and society as a whole. This approach became known as 'disability management'. Disability management, unabashedly embracing the belief that society values work, has continued to focus on finding solutions to disability issues within the context of the workplace. Initially the focus was on temporary disabilities resulting from injury or illness, usually as a result of employment. However, this quickly expanded to include all acquired disabilities regardless of aetiology and is now expanding to include all issues of disability that impact on a person's ability to live a full and independent life embracing work and all the activities of daily living.

REFERENCES

Akabas S 1986 Disability management: a longstanding trade union mission with some new initiatives. Journal of Applied Rehabilitation Counseling 17(3):33–37

Anderson T 1975 An alternative frame of reference for rehabilitation: the helping process versus the medical model. Archives of Physical Medicine and Rehabilitation 56:101–104

Berkowitz E, McQuaid K 1980 Welfare reform in the 1950s. Social Service Review 54:45–58

Blaxter M 1975 Disability and rehabilitation: some questions of definition. In: Cox C M, Mead A (eds) A Sociology of Medical Practice. Macmillan, New York, pp 207–223

Canadian Human Rights Code 1980 http://laws.justice.gc.ca/en/h-6/31147.html

Galton F 1901 The possible improvement of the human breed under the existing conditions of law and sentiment. Man 1(132):161–164

Galton F 1904 Eugenics. Its definition, scope and aims. The American Journal of Sociology 10:1–6

Galvin D 1986 Health promotion, disability management and rehabilitation in the workplace. Rehabilitation Literature 47(9–10):218–223

Garland R 1995 The Eye of the Beholder: Deformity and disability in the Graeco-Roman world. Cornell University Press, Ithaca, NY

Habeck R V, Scully S M, Van Tol B et al 1998 Successful employer strategies for preventing and managing disability. Rehabilitation Counseling Bulletin 42(2):144–161

Hahn R A, Kleinman A 1983 Biomedical practice and anthropological theory: frameworks and directions. Annual Review of Anthropology 12:305–333

Hershenson D 2000 Toward a cultural anthropology of disability and rehabilitation. Rehabilitation Counseling Bulletin 43(3):150–159

Hogg-Johnson S, Cole D 2003 Early prognostic factors for duration on benefits among workers with compensated occupational soft tissue injuries. Occupational and Environmental Medicine 60:240–256

Jarvikoski A, Lahelma E 1980 Early Rehabilitation at the Work Place. World Rehabilitation Fund, New York, p 79

Kudlick C 2003 Review essay. Disability history: why we need another 'other'. American Historical Review 3:763–793

McCarthy H 2003 The disability rights movement: experiences and perspectives of selected leaders in the disability community. Rehabilitation Counseling Bulletin 46(4):209–223

Mitchell K 2002 Best practices for creating an effective return-to-work program. Compensation and Benefits Management 18(3):34–37

Nagi S 1969 Disability and Rehabilitation: Legal, clinical, and self-concepts and measurement. Ohio State University Press, Ohio

Otlowski M F A, Williamson R 2003 Ethical and legal issues and the 'new genetics'. The Medical Journal of Australia 178(11):582–585

Richards M 2004 Perfecting people: selective breeding at the Oneida Community (1869–1879) and the Eugenics Movement. New Genetics and Society 23(1):47–71

Rubin S E, Pusch B D, Fogerty C et al 1995 Enhancing the cultural sensitivity of rehabilitation counsellors. Rehabilitation Education 9:253–264

Schwartz G 1984 Disability costs: the impeding crisis. Business and Health 1(6):25–28

Stein H E 1979 Rehabilitation and chronic illness in American culture. The cultural psychodynamics of medical and social problems. Journal of Psychological Anthropology 2:153–176

US Rehabilitation Act 1973 http://www.webaim.org/coordination/law/us/504/ and http://www.disabilityresources.org/REHAB-ACT.html

Van Hooser J R, Rice D B 1989 Disability Management in the Workplace. The National Institute on Rehabilitation Issues, Savannah, GA

World Health Organization 1981 Disability Prevention and Rehabilitation. Report of the WHO expert committee on disability prevention and rehabilitation. World Health Organization Technical Report Series 668. World Health Organization, Geneva

Chapter 2

Components of disability management

LEARNING OBJECTIVES

■ Overview of the essential disability management components
■ Understand the various components of the disability management process

INTRODUCTION

The practice of disability management (DM) has evolved over the past few decades and there is no disputing its positive intentions. It is an interesting field as it deals with a corporation's planned interventions as associated with all components of its business and expenses, including the area of occupational and non-occupational disability. It also encompasses the entire spectrum of health for individuals and the psychosocial interactions of individuals and their potential responses to disability.

Disability management includes several key components:

■ data analysis
■ the disability programme design (prevention, claim initiation, claims management, case management, return to regular work, return to transitional work and rehabilitation)
■ recognition of its importance by senior management
■ the measuring of results.

This chapter will provide a brief overview of these components, then future chapters will expand on each of these essential topics.

Consider the following scenario to emphasize why prevention, claim initiation, claims management, case management, return to regular work, return to transitional work and rehabilitation components are an important factor in the DM programme. Imagine Joe, an average citizen – he smokes less than a packet of cigarettes a day and has a demanding job that has him working from 7 am to 6 pm every day, which means leaving home at 5:30 am to beat the traffic. He has two children with a variety of 'programmes' to run to every night including football, dance and guitar lessons. His wife works full-time in an equally responsible job. She drops the kids off in the morning at school and Joe has to be home to pick them up by 6 pm every day then start running them to their various activities. Somewhere on the run during the day he has a coffee and doughnut, and then a bag of crisps for lunch with a cola and cigarette (while running from meeting to meeting) then, during the evening, he picks up a McDonald's from a drive-through with the kids on their way to activities. He has not had time to exercise and is a little overweight, struggling occasionally with high blood pressure.

Joe tries to get to the doctor for a yearly check-up but has not been in over two years, other than taking the kids to the clinic when they need to get antibiotics for various ear infections or other childhood ailments. Trying to get home one evening he is running late and distracted. He runs a yellow light, and is 'broadsided' by a truck. The car is written off and Joe is hospitalized with a broken shoulder, facial cuts and a broken leg. He is discharged from the hospital after two days with instructions to come back for cast removal in four weeks. Joe is unable to return to work (RTW) due to the pain and immobility; he is struggling, trying to figure out how to replace the car as he had cancelled the collision coverage on the vehicle the previous year to reduce the insurance costs so that he could afford to send his son to a tutor twice a week. He is wondering how they will pay all the bills without his income.

Joe thinks he remembers something about his employer having a short-term disability insurance benefit but he is having some difficulty getting anyone in Human Resources to call him back. He finally gets some forms in the mail from the company to fill out and send back. Two months into his disability a cheque arrives from the insurance company but it is significantly less than what he had expected. A note is attached to the effect that additional medical information will need to be submitted prior to any additional cheque being issued. The bills are starting to pile up quickly and the pain in his shoulder is excruciating at times. Joe realizes the disability payment is not even half his usual salary due to the maximum on the plan and starts to panic about paying bills. He has not heard from anyone at work and starts worrying about the status of his job when he is ready to return to work. He worked hard when he was there and does not understand why the workplace has not called. No one at work seems to care and his supervisor is not calling. It feels as though his work contributions were not as valued as he thought. Joe gets the cast off his leg and starts physiotherapy twice a week; however, he is still struggling with the intense pain in his shoulder and is still not completely mobile. He needs plastic surgery on one of the cuts on his face – it was very deep and is healing in a crooked line. The scar is so severe Joe feels it is causing people to look at him in public places. He spends most of his time lying in bed. His wife is becoming increasingly frustrated with having to do all of the running with the kids and chores while Joe isolates himself in the house. He develops pneumonia due to his immobility and, perhaps, in part due to the increased number of cigarettes he has been smoking since he has been off work. Joe is readmitted to hospital for intense antibiotic treatment. In this scenario it is impossible to separate the personal, work interaction and disability factors.

Now let's look at the same case but from the perspective of a company with a solid DM programme in place. The company has set up a variety of health-promotion programmes and has a gym with on-site programmes that run during lunch hours to assist employees in reducing risk factors and supports healthy balanced lifestyles. If Joe had been with this company, within a day of the accident the workplace would provide information about the disability programme and procedures. Joe would receive reassurance from his supervisor that the workload is covered on a temporary basis and let him know they look forward to when he can return to work. This demonstrates that the employer cares and is anxious to see Joe return to work. The DM practitioner – either internal or external – would contact Joe to determine if he needed any assistance with the healthcare system and his recovery, and would ensure that Joe is aware that the workplace is committed to assisting him to return to work as soon as possible. The case manager would have solid connections in the medical and social community to assist in facilitating appropriate care. Joe would be provided with support as the disability progressed, ensuring that therapy commenced as soon as possible on his shoulder and leg. He would be encouraged to stop into work, if possible, for a visit at the worksite to maintain the connection. Perhaps some possible modified work would be explored during the recovery period. The workplace and Joe would be clear on the RTW projected timelines and activities that surround that expected date of return.

DISABILITY MANAGEMENT CONTINUUM

In commencing a DM programme it is important to understand the starting position of the corporation by establishing a baseline through data analysis. This will assist in quantifying the value of the programme, measuring the results and looking for areas of continuous improvement.

In addition, a statistical baseline can assist in establishing the financial impact for employers to drive management support for the DM programme. This will also demonstrate the value of the programme from an employee-retention and workplace-of-choice perspective (Fig. 2.1).

Data analysis

Good data analysis at the start of a programme can assist in the identification of trends and programme needs. A substantial amount of information can be collected and analysed to achieve smooth appropriate planning, programme implementation and programme evaluation. The function of data analysis is to organize, summarize and present the information in a useful

Figure 2.1 The disability management continuum.

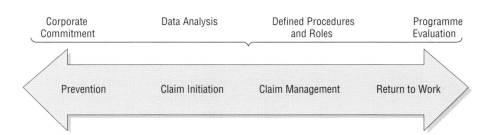

format to develop and maintain the programme. A detailed report on existing conditions and service provides an important base. It assists in quantifying the concerns and successes, and determines the priorities that should be addressed in the programme. Data analysis also identifies areas that require more information to establish accurately the needs of an organization.

The best time to start data analysis is prior to the programme development. A quantitative and qualitative baseline evaluation will ensure the right areas are focused on and will avoid designing programmes that do not meet the workplace needs.

Take, for example, a worksite that puts in a back injury prevention programme to address workers' compensation costs. Unfortunately, in reviewing the data, 60% of the costs and injuries were from knee concerns. Therefore the lack of analysis of data resulted in a programme being put in place that would not address the primary issues.

Qualitative areas that can be examined are employee attitudes, interest and opinions. These evaluations can be carried out with focus groups or brief surveys.

Quantitative areas that can be examined for the collection of data include workers' compensation data, sick leave or short-term disability data, and long-term disability data. Additionally, data from the Employee Assistance Plan or the Drug Plan can be used for some predictive trending. In some circumstances other excused-leave programmes such as the emergency days under the Employment Standards Act in Canada or the Family Medical Leave Act in the USA may be captured.

It is important when collecting information that the baseline data collection with standardized measures is consistent. The Washington Business Group on Health (WBGH) Council on Employee Health and Productivity released standard metrics in June 2003. These metrics define clear parameters on cost per employee, cost per claim, cost as a percentage of payroll, lost days per 100 employees, average claim duration, claim incidence and RTW efficiency. These data can all be documented as solid quantifiable costs.

Cost per employee

As defined in the WBGH (2003) document the cost per employee represents 'the benefits paid, per benefit category, during a given time period, divided by the average number of employees eligible for benefits during the same time period'.

Average cost of claim

'The average cost per claim for a given period is calculated by dividing the total claim payments made during a given period by the number of claims open at some point during the period. An open claim is defined as a claim for which benefits were paid at some point during a specified period' (WBGH 2003).

Costs as a percentage of payroll

Total benefits paid divided by the total payroll costs of employees eligible for the benefit.

Lost days per 100 employees

Lost time days multiplied by the total number of hours worked divided by 200 000 will produce the lost days per 100 employees.

Average claim duration

The duration of the claim is the interval in calendar days between the day an individual first becomes unable to work due to illness or injury and the date the claim ends.

Claim incidence

Claim incidence is also known as claim frequency. It is the number of claims that occur per 100 employees and is calculated by taking the total number of claims multiplied by 200 000 (number of hours worked by 100 employees in a year) then divided by the total hours worked.

Return-to-work efficiency

This refers to the speed and type of RTW, i.e. how many employees have returned to regular duties, how many to modified duties in order to transition back to their regular job, how many to permanently altered jobs and how many to alternative jobs outside their home or workplace? Of those that returned on modified duties, how long was the programme and what was the result? (Establish the following factors, then measure how quickly these goals are achieved.)

Each of these categories can be broken down by division location, department and shift. The data analysis could also include the demographics of the workforce, including age, gender, years of service and number of previous claims. If an employer has multiple sites, any applicable legislative restrictions should be documented and noted. This is to continue to recognize the impact of external influences on the illness and injury behaviour.

An example of how legislation can have a profound impact on behaviour can be found in the RTW provisions under the Ontario Workplace Safety and Insurance Board (WSIB) legislation. This provides significant incentive and penalties to employers and employees if they do not participate in early and safe return to work. Ultimately this legislation changed behaviour dramatically with the duration of claims decreasing from 17.8 in 1993 to 14.3 in 2002 (WSIB 2002). This does not ensure that the RTW is appropriate; it simply ensures that the injured worker is back at work so that the additional metric of success of return to regular work can show the results of the programme.

Historical data provide a solid base on which to build the programme. It is essential to establish ongoing revisiting of the baseline to determine the needs for any additional programmes, to make sure that the developed programmes are addressing the needs and in order to communicate the results.

DISABILITY MANAGEMENT PROGRAMME DESIGN

Disability management programme design can be based on the analysis of needs and current understanding of essential elements of DM programmes. Specific goals and objectives need to be established based on workplace needs. It is important that DM initiatives are in line with the corporation's overall objectives and mandate. The components of the programme include all the important elements of prevention, claim initiation, claims/case management, RTW and accommodation. Additional details of policies, procedures, and roles and responsibilities can be found in Chapter 6.

Prevention

Society understands the importance of healthy lifestyles and prevention. Personal nutrition, adequate exercise, not smoking, drinking moderately and dealing with issues as they arise are all important elements in decreasing the incidence of disability. Work safety practices, ergonomics, employee training and minimizing workplace hazards all assist in the prevention of needless incidents (Wilson & McCutcheon 2003).

Prevention programmes can be very effective in the workplace. It is one of the few places where there is a captive audience and a consistent peer group that can reinforce positive lifestyle choices. As discussed in Elswick (2002), Chevron-Texaco has sustained smoking reduction from 28% to 18%, sustained a two-year recovery rate from substance abuse at 70%, reduced occupational incidents by 50% and reduced occupational incidents with lost time by 60%. Regular fitness centre participants had 71% lower inpatient experiences and 26% lower drug expenditures than non-participants. The projected return on investment is US$6.9 million per year. The results of health promotion programmes have positive longterm effects.

Prevention programmes can include everything from internal health promotion to targeted health and safety initiatives to external employee assistance programmes. Ultimately the best way to determine prevention programmes is to look at the needs of the employees, the disability data, the drug utilization data and the common trends, then design the programmes that will address the greatest need.

Early identification

The creation of 'day one' reporting for all absences is essential. The employer should set the expectation to return to work from the start. In Cole et al (2002) it is clearly demonstrated that the expectation to return to work made a significant difference in durations of absences. Of course, it is not sufficient to just report and monitor: there must also be an element of management of these absences.

The early identification of employees who need assistance is very important. It can prevent an employee, prior to a medical condition, from becoming disabled. It allows intervention to ensure that employees are receiving the right care before any crisis occurs. Imagine a man who has occasional pain in his upper neck as he sits at the computer terminal every day. If he simply tolerates the pain day after day and does not seek ergonomic adjustments to his workstation or if he does not pursue any healthcare treatment he will progress to increasing levels of pain and eventual disability. The longer the pain continues without intervention the more difficult the treatment and recovery will be. Early intervention also assists in conveying the attitude that the company cares about its employees' health as it relates to performing the daily task. This is clearly one of the most important periods in a claim. Disability management practitioners, through initial interventions, can make a profound difference to the outcomes of a claim.

A study by Gatchet et al (2003) clearly demonstrated greater cost savings associated with early intervention. The results further identified that 'high risk subjects who received early intervention displayed statistically significant fewer incidents of chronic pain disability on a wide range of work, healthcare utilization, medication use, and self report pain variables'.

Another compelling example of positive workplace intervention is recognizing elements in the work environment that may be causing psychosocial incongruence. A change in management philosophy can create uncertainties in the employee groups. Attention needs to be given to the positive introduction of change. The change management process should include communication. As discussed in Kotter (1996) communication is one of the underpinnings of successful change: 'major change is usually impossible unless most employees are willing to help, often to the point of making short term sacrifices'. Poorly managed change can result in unhappy and uncertain employees. A well-run organization with good communication strategies will have healthier employees.

Claim and case management

A DM programme needs a strong element of claim and case management. This consists of the activities that ensure that when an employee is off work he or she is receiving optimal healthcare and focusing on recovery. This may also be viewed as the period where service coordination occurs.

Claim management is different from case management. Claim management can be summarized as the evidence required to administer the claim. Is there sufficient medical documentation to support the absence? Is there continuing information to support the absence? Is there a RTW date? Are there documented capabilities and limitations to facilitate early and safe RTW?

The case-management component of the programme focuses on activities that occur in the period when the employee is off work. This may include assisting the employee to become involved with the right treatment. It should determine if the employee is being treated appropriately, if the employee is satisfied with treatment, and whether or not that treatment will result in recovery. As stated by Jane Vos (2004), Vice-President of Organizational Solutions, 'Employees often need assistance finding their way through the healthcare maze and we help them through that enhancing recovery and ultimately facilitating RTW much earlier'. It is the essential time to become involved prior to the disability mindset starting. Interventions do not stop at appropriate treatment needs as lost time can encompass employee and employer perceptions of disability. Consider a worker who has a serious and significant injury – such as an acquired brain injury following a vehicle accident – which will lead to a lengthy recovery and will very likely result in permanent changes to capabilities. The longer the employee is off work the more intense the feelings of not belonging become. It is essential that the workplace remains supportive and for the treatment to focus on restoring the employee to optimal function.

In studies going back to the beginning of the DM era it has been found that even casual contact with the employee decreases absence by 30% (Bigos et al 1991). Of course DM has grown in sophistication but the underlying principle of staying in touch has not changed.

Aspects of both of these functions can be managed internally at the employer if they have appropriately qualified regulated healthcare professional staff or handled by an external agency such as a Third Party Administrator. Case management can be performed effectively (internally or externally) as long as the process is defined and appropriately managed. Large corporations may have in-house case managers. The advantage of the internal approach is the familiarity with the workplace and constant access to supervisors and the management team for a quick response to policy changes. The disadvantage is that benefit decisions are then retained at the company and can be affected by issues other than just the disability. Additionally, confidentiality may be a concern when case management is performed internally. The advantage of an external firm includes the fact that DM is their core competency. This is what they specialize in and the staff will have expertise and access to DM resources that internal staff may not have. An experienced firm has insight from their book of business and can assist in ensuring best practice. It is also advantageous to delegate the authority to accept or deny claims based on sufficient medical documentation and treatment plans to an external source that has clear acceptance criteria used on their book of business. Another advantage is the protection of confidential medical information as it minimizes the information flowing through a company administrator. It is important to emphasize that, whether managed internally or externally, confidentiality is compulsory. Sensitive medical information should not be shared inappropriately; informed consents are essential and mandatory in a good DM programme. Limitations and capabilities are necessary components that can be shared at the employer level to assist with the RTW process.

Green-McKenzie et al (1998) found a 41–59% reduction in indemnity payments and a 46–67% reduction in lost-time cases, which were realized after the healthcare management initiative was fully in place. Additionally, they found that cost-control measures without comprehensive case management did not decrease these parameters significantly. The parameters of the healthcare management programme included implementation of an early and safe RTW programme, assistance with scheduling of specialist appointments and coordination of the process flow of information between providers (workers' compensation, healthcare providers) and supervisors, implementation of a close follow-up system and the institution of in-house administration of all legal cases.

It is essential to realize that each individual and each workplace is different, and that responses to disability are a complex interplay of workplace factors, family, external influences such as support systems, prior experiences, treatment availability and other elements as discussed in Chapter 3.

Additionally, it is important to realize that when an employee becomes ill and is trying to get through the healthcare process, he or she may be particularly overwhelmed and vulnerable. In research conducted by Gates (2000) participants indicated that the support of the case manager was a primary reason for RTW.

The DM practitioner's (case manager) role is often seen as one of a liaison in the system. The DM practitioner has the primary objective of assisting the employee to overcome blocks to recovery and RTW. Disability management may involve activities such as coordinating services outside the workplace with healthcare providers, community agencies, and organizing activities inside the workplace with supervisors, co-workers and union representatives.

As soon as possible following an absence, the DM practitioner should make contact with the employee to let them know about the DM programme and the support that is available to them during this time.

The next important element in the DM process is the monitoring of the physical recovery/treatment process. Prompt and appropriate care has been identified as one of the key variables in recovery (Adams & Williams 2003, Baril et al 2003, Shaw et al 2002). The DM practitioner would ensure that physical treatment is proceeding. This does not mean that DM practitioners take the place of physicians – they simply ensure that there are no systemic delays preventing timely and appropriate treatment.

Disability management programmes often involve pulling together resources dispersed in the workplace and community to bring the employee back to work. This role needs to be performed by a professional with specific DM skills, as discussed in Chapter 6.

One objective is to obtain capabilities as soon as possible and focus on appropriate and timely RTW. It may include an independent medical evaluation or function ability evaluation if there is a need to quantify capabilities beyond the treating healthcare provider's assessment capabilities. One possible tool in the DM process is the independent medical examination (IME) or the function ability evaluation (FAE). These can be useful tools if designed to answer specific questions and if they focus on positive outcomes. It is not sufficient to obtain an IME or FAE to determine what is wrong with the employee; it is most important to ensure that part of the assessment will look at potential methods of resolution.

Catastrophic cases will require a different skill set and multiple professionals to design suitable action plans than those required for less serious injuries or illnesses.

Return to work

Return to work is a primary goal of any DM programme. In order to effectively return an employee to work the essential duties of the job must be known. If required, arrange for a Job Demands Analysis to understand fully the parameters of the job duties. Speak with the employee, the supervisor and union personnel (if applicable) to acquire an accurate picture of the job.

Once an employee is off work, discussions should start with the person regarding their RTW; it is important to state the RTW expectation as soon as the employee is off work. As discussed in Shaw et al (2002) the individual's personal meaning of disability and RTW is very relevant. It is essential to shape the individual's expectation toward RTW. Emphasizing transition back to the regular job is the objective whenever possible.

Once the RTW becomes imminent a determination needs to be made as to whether the return will require transitional work, accommodation, alternate placement or retraining. It is necessary to explore fully the individual's cognitive or physical capabilities as compared to the job demands. Some caution must be used in this process, particularly when it comes to pre-existing conditions which may not have been taken into account upon hire but may undermine the RTW process if capabilities are reviewed outside the actual injury or illness.

Once the capabilities have been established, a meeting with the worksite and worker may need to take place. If the employee is simply returning to a regular position a meeting may not be required. If there is any transitional nature to the RTW a meeting should be established to review all aspects of the RTW process, to ensure that all parties understand their respective roles, and to establish the process for follow-up to ensure successful reintegration into the workplace. A RTW plan should include a summary of capabilities and be developed with specific timelines for progress back to a regular job.

It is important for health and safety to be considered in the reintegration of the employee to the worksite. Explain the safety provisions of the position and identify who to go to for help if there are any questions. It is also essential to consider the safety of others when placing an employee back to work – the employee should be able to perform the job in a manner that does not endanger other workers.

Many people are very nervous when they return to work and these fears can be reduced by defining the expectations then setting the plan in place. Return-to-work progress needs to be monitored to ensure appropriate transition back into the workplace. Return to work may require the intervention of a specialist such as an occupational therapist, physiotherapist, ergonomist, occupational health nurse or other professionals to identify elements of the RTW that may create barriers if not addressed properly. The fit between the worker's capabilities and the job is an essential component of RTW. The DM practitioner should stay in frequent contact with both the worker and the immediate supervisor until the worker has moved back to a regular position. If problems arise, the interventions should be immediate to resolve difficulties and preserve the RTW plan. Follow-up in two-week intervals to ensure that everything stays on course and that the worker stays at work.

It is also important to have a formal closure meeting to celebrate the success of transition back to regular duties and bring closure to the plan.

Safe and timely RTW programmes are a reality that demonstrate significant favourable human and financial results. Curtis and Scott (2004) document the positive impact of RTW. The workplace must be prepared to promote transitional jobs for returning workers who may have temporary limitations in functioning. If it identified early that the employee will not be able to return to a regular job in the workplace due to the severity of the condition then rehabilitation should be considered and interventions looked at early in the process before the disability mindset takes hold.

PROGRAMME DEVELOPMENT AND EVALUATION

The final but key element to a successful DM programme is to measure and document its success. In the design of successful DM programmes, goals and objectives would be established to provide the basis for measurement of success. Programme evaluation is important to address areas of continuous improvement, which have become part of the social fabric of business, and DM programmes should integrate prevention information into a company's strategic and project planning processes.

CONCLUSION

Disability management programmes implemented with the above key considerations will decrease the human and financial cost of disabilities. The key areas include data analysis, solid programme design, prevention, claim initiation, claims and case management, RTW and continuous improvement. All programmes require senior management support and should be measured to demonstrate effectiveness and a return on investment.

REFERENCES

Adams J H, Williams A 2003 What affects return to work for graduates of a pain management programme with chronic upper limb pain. Journal of Occupational Rehabilitation 13(2):91–106

Baril R, Berthelette D, Massicotte P 2003 Early return to work of injured workers: multidimensional patterns of individual and organizational factors. Safety Science 41: 277–300

Bigos S J, Battie M C, Spengler D M et al 1991 A prospective study of work perceptions and psychosocial factors affecting the report of back injury. Spine 16(1):1–6

Cole D C, Mondloch M V, Hogg-Johnson S for the Early Claimant Cohort Prognostic Modelling Group 2002 Listening to injured workers: how recovery expectations predict outcomes – a prospective study. Canadian Medical Association Journal 166(6):749–754

Curtis J, Scott L 2004 Integrating disability management into strategic plans. American Association of Occupational Health Nurses Journal 52(7):298–301
http://www.aaohn.org/practice/journal/index.cfm

Elswick J 2002 Employers cite success with disability programs. Employee Benefit News, December http://www.benefitnews.com/detail.cfm?id=3842&terms=|elswick|

Gatchet R J, Polatin P B, Noe C et al 2003 Treatment and cost-effectiveness of early intervention for acute low back pain patients: a one-year prospective study. Journal of Occupational Rehabilitation 13(1):1–9

Gates L B 2000 Workplace accommodation as a social process. Journal of Occupational Rehabilitation 10(1):85–98

Green-McKenzie J, Parkerson S, Bernacki E 1998 Comparison of workers' compensation costs for two cohorts of injured workers before and after the introduction of managed care. Journal of Occupational Medicine 40(6):568–572

Kotter J P 1996 Leading Change. Harvard Business School Press, Boston, MA

Shaw L, Segal R, Polatjkos H et al 2002 Understanding return to work behaviors: promoting the importance of individual perceptions in the study of return to work. Disability and Rehabilitation 44(4):185–195

Vos J 2004 Personal communication. Organizational Solutions, Burlington, Ontario

Washington Business Group on Health 2004 www.wbgh.org

Wilson L, McCutcheon D 2003 Industrial Safety and Risk Management. The University of Alberta Press, Edmonton, Alberta

Workplace Safety and Insurance Board of Ontario 2002 http://www.wsib.on.ca/ar2002_home_e.htm

Chapter 3

A conceptual model for disability management

LEARNING OBJECTIVES

- Understand the basis for a conceptual model in disability management
- Describe the variety of influencers on disability outcomes
- Recognize that disability management addresses the individual as part of the broader social system

INTRODUCTION

Disability management (DM) is an emerging discipline in which the contribution to the corporation and its employees is important to the financial and human reduction of costs. As with any emerging profession, critical thought needs to be applied to the order and semblance of the task, principles, practices and facts that govern the profession and make the interventions successful and easy to replicate. The knowledge base of a profession evolves and a complex interplay of forces over time shapes the activities. The profession has a mandate to meet a basic need of society and has gathered recognition through their ability to impact the overall status of social problems (resolution of a social issue) and input on the corporation's bottom line. Specialized knowledge allows practitioners in the field to use specific applications that define and guide decisions to make this type of contribution.

Most people have views of the world, their work and the subject of their work, in this case DM. The beliefs give direction to people who work in the occupation. These beliefs form the 'theory' of their lives. In this chapter we will introduce a theoretical model that is constructed from DM philosophies and beliefs about 'work' gathered from current knowledge and beliefs, as present in academia and the workplace.

'A theory may be defined as a scientifically acceptable general principle which governs practice or is proposed to explain observed facts. Another definition of theory is that it is a logical interconnected set of propositions used to describe, explain, and predict a part of the empirical world' (Riehl & Roy 1980: 3). Theories are proposals which give a reasonable explanation of an event. They are ideas about how or why something happens in the manner in which it occurs.

A model can be defined as 'a symbolic depiction in logical terms of an idealized, relatively simple situation showing the structure of the original system' (Hazzard & Kergin 1971 from Riehl & Roy 1980: 6). A model is a conceptual representation of reality, not reality itself but an illustration, a shell of the features within a discipline that give direction to the cluster of informal rules that are formulated to guide the profession. An example of a model is the miniature replica of new buildings that often sit under a glass case in the lobby during the design and building phase of a construction project. These are not the real thing but a model that is used to emulate the structure and demonstrate how the finished product will look.

A model is systematically constructed, scientifically based and logically related to sets of concepts that identify the logical and essential components of DM practice. The parts are related to each other through a cohesive and systematic approach.

The basis for this DM model comprises the underpinnings of social sciences systems theory. First proposed by Ludwig von Bertalanfy, a biologist in the 1940s, general systems theory represents an effort to provide a comprehensive theoretical model embracing all living systems and applicable to all the behavioural sciences. Bertalanfy's major contribution was to provide a framework for looking at seemingly unrelated phenomena to understand how together they represent interrelated components of a larger system. A system is a complex assembly of component parts which are in mutual interaction. 'Nothing and nobody exist in isolation; the world is made up of systems within systems. Open, living systems exist by virtue of their interaction with the environment. They constantly change' (Goldenberg & Goldenberg 1980).

Our conceptual model portrays a systematic view of the field of DM. It describes the key terms and relationships between concepts, goal and interventions. Models include three basic components: beliefs and values; goals of practice/what we want to achieve; and knowledge and skills required to obtain the goals.

PRACTICE = BELIEFS + GOALS + KNOWLEDGE

BELIEFS AND VALUES

Occupations and individuals formulate beliefs about how humans behave under given circumstances. People do not live in isolation but interact with many other things in the community and in society itself. Therefore any profession dealing with humans must have some understanding of how people, or the recipients of their services, function and interrelate with the world around them.

Values play a strong role in shaping the collective vision of a profession. The practice of DM is still fairly early in its evolution, and the knowledge base leaves ample room for uncertainty around the practice parameters. The absence of 100% defined knowledge means that values are important guides for practice. As the base of knowledge grows, values will have a significant impact on the direction and will influence the practice dramatically.

Deeply ingrained in DM practice is a belief that each person's individuality and 'humanism' is essential and has worth regardless of the impairment. This is emphasized by strong desire of the profession to focus on the capabilities and assets of the individual. There is the recognition that each person has a set of experiences and desires that serve as the background on which they formulate their decisions and actions. The values include the recognition that disability is individualistic and that each experience is unique to the individual. No potential ability or residual capability is too small or insignificant. Part of the DM practitioner's job is to ensure that capacity is identified and used when resolving the disability. There is potential in every person, sometimes unrecognized but there is potential.

It is essential to maintain hope in the face of unfavourable odds and deteriorating conditions. It can also be said that an understanding exists that determination and individual commitment of the individuals to take an active role in their own success is critical to the success of DM strategies. This concept is in direct opposition to the passive 'patient' approach that proliferates in the medical model.

Disability management practitioners need to recognize that there is a huge range of individual differences that must be taken into consideration when applying any model or theory to treatment and interventions.

GOALS

The occupational group of disability managers needs to agree on the common purpose of their interventions. It is also important that the client (i.e. the ill or injured employee) needs to be clear about the parameters of the DM practitioner's role.

The traditional goal of DM practice is to return the disabled individual to work/function. This definition continues to evolve to encompass the ensuring of appropriate interventions during the period of disability. As we expand the definition to 'comprehensive disability management', the programme focus shifts to assisting the individual to obtain appropriate care and recover to optimal function and ultimately return to work (RTW). Disability management stresses the importance and recognizes the influences on the worker that directly impact on the outcomes. Additionally, it focuses on the need for feeding all information gleaned from dealing with the illness or injury of the worker back to a central point of contact: the DM practitioner. In order to learn from experiences and prevent the recurrence of injury or illness, knowledge of successful interventions must be assimilated and used to continually improve the practice area. The DM professionals must operate within the legal and regulatory guidelines when performing all components of their role.

Within the goals of the DM model there is a basic understanding that humans have an occupational nature, that 'work' is an essential part of human life and that the centrality of work is an essential part of human welfare (Frese & Mohr 1987, Winefield et al 1991).

KNOWLEDGE

Once a profession has identified the extent of the knowledge, in this case surrounding the disability and DM, a definition of the knowledge requirement becomes possible. The acquisition of technical knowledge required to function effectively as a DM practitioner surrounds the understanding that this is a profession grounded in the belief that humans are biological creatures who can be affected by injury and disease. The intervention goal, which encompasses assisting individuals, is based on individuals' returning to functioning optimally, and to RTW following a disabling event.

THE MODEL

The model conceptualizes the workplace from the worker's point of view. The model has three major spheres: work; the internal workplace; and the non-workplace external environment. These spheres are permeable, recognizing the interconnectedness of multiple components. The system has a tendency to have a steady state or balance. When the balance is altered the other components move in and out.

Every conceptual model should describe the key terms and relationships between concepts, goals and interventions. The model is a systematic view where the elements of each key component and influence are clearly delineated to clarify the interactions of the model. Overlap among the elements is recognized.

PHILOSOPHY

The DM practitioner within the comprehensive DM process facilitates early and safe RTW and strives to decrease the human and financial costs of disabilities regardless of the employee's age, gender, ethnicity, and culture or health status. The DM practitioner accomplishes this through expertise and practice, blended with collaboration, education and empowerment of the workplace community.

In a comprehensive DM programme the practitioner is responsive to work, workplace parties and external influences. The need to understand the critical importance of these interactions and their influence on the worker and the worksite led to the development of the model.

DESCRIPTION

The multidimensional scope of DM is represented in the elements within the inner circle and within the broader circle. The workplace is analogous with the workers, management, co-workers, and the union if present. This environment is influenced by the individual and collective attitudes of workers, co-workers, union and management participants. Interplay occurs among these elements of the work environment. Being able to understand the needs of these varied and complex roles leads to successful comprehensive DM. A workplace is simply a designated facility or area where work is performed; it must comply with legislation, standards and laws. Addi-

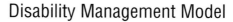

Figure 3.1 The disability management model.

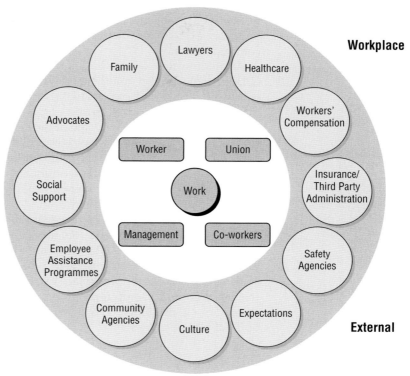

tionally, the workplace will have policies, procedures and philosophy that govern the organization's actions. Some workplaces create an environment with unique physical and mental stressors. These elements need to be recognized and addressed because if left unattended they can create an organization susceptible to poor DM practices.

The workplace realm is bordered by dotted lines indicating ongoing and fluid relationships with interactions inside and outside this sphere (Fig. 3.1). The outer circle represents elements that may or may not interact with the work elements within the inside circle. The workplace is not a self-contained environment holding the employees captive 24 hours a day, so we need to recognize the interactions with providers, suppliers, customers, family and community.

The outer circle represents elements that may have an influence on the worker. These are multiple and include healthcare providers, Workers' Compensation Board or insurers or third-party administrators, safety agencies, expectations, culture, community agencies, employee assistance programmes, social support, advocates, family, lawyers and healthcare itself. The outer elements are important and the impacts of these relationships need to be considered in the comprehensive DM process. Ignoring the influence of the outer circle will significantly reduce the outcome of the DM efforts. The workplace can influence these elements and interrelationships by the selection and use of appropriate preferred providers for treatment, resolution of disability, and other issues impacting disability. A level of trust needs to be established with workers so that they do not feel the necessity to pursue external legal representation. One method of doing this is through communication.

An interesting example is in a workplace that had a high propensity to obtain legal counsel following a workplace incident. Management and employee representatives created a short and easy-to-understand communication that was posted on the employee information bulletin board. It demonstrated the financial value of the claim with and without legal representation. The workplace was located in a state that had a cap on permanent impairment awards so the intervention of lawyers in fact reduced the overall monies that the worker ultimately received. Once the employees were aware of the facts they were less likely to pursue legal representation following work-related incidents.

This model also conveys the necessity of work being the central element. The interactions throughout the model indicate participative roles and responsibilities in active DM. The outer elements are important and the impacts of these relationships need to be considered in the DM process. In some circumstances the workplace can influence these interrelationships by the selection and use of appropriate preferred partners for treatment and resolution of disability. The interrelationships should be prioritized for optimal DM outcomes.

Key definitions

Work

The workplace internal environment refers to the distinct features that can comprise a work setting. Interplay also occurs among elements of this environment. Results of the interactions ultimately describe the workplace and the workers' experience of working. The internal environment is influenced by several elements, particularly the corporate mission.

An important role of the DM practitioner in the workplace environment is to facilitate the placement of workers according to their physical, mental and emotional capacities. The goal is to allow workers to perform the required work with an optimal degree of efficiency and without endangering their own health and safety or that of others. Teamwork is vital to the success of this model. A successful workplace DM programme builds a team commitment to encourage the worker to actively participate in seeking health, recovery and RTW. No single worker in an organization is responsible for DM and returning the employee to work safely. Workplaces with successfully implemented DM have defined roles and responsibilities for all team members (Tate et al 1999).

Work is the centre of the model as its premise is based on the knowledge that work is central to life. Work is in fact a complete facet of all community life. Societies are made possible and function through the division of labour and the integration of various forms of work. Everyone is interdependent on the productivity of others. Kielhoner (1992) states that 'participation in occupation has an impact on the individual's biological and psychological health. Occupation is essential to the well-being of the individual'. It is widely documented that individuals have a psychological need for occupation (Feather & Bond 1983, Jones & Davis 1991, Pearlin & Liberman 1979). The occupation motive emerges from the biologically and culturally based desires to engage in activity to discover and create and to realize a degree of mastery (Heider 1958, Kelley 1967, Pearlin & Liberman 1979). Through work people are able to discover new information and potentials for action, experience control, develop confidence and reaffirm their self-worth. Occupation is recognized as having a role in creating, affirming and experiencing meaning in life (Dooley & Catalano 1988, Winegardner et al 1984). Many examples can be found where the absence of work has led to a downward spiral of functioning as a contributing member of society and has resulted in difficult psychological effects to the individual.

To be effective the DM practitioner must acknowledge human variables and the multiple influence of the work environment. It is essential to work as an active team member committed to overcoming potential workplace barriers to successful RTW. It is recognized that the 'worlds' of work and non-work are vitally interconnected. It can be recognized and understood that the effects of increased demands placed on workers by contemporary society need to be addressed. In so doing, such practitioners are better able to develop programmes that are useful and effective. The authors are optimistic that in spite of the complexities inherent in optimal RTW at the workplace a 'fair–fair' situation for both employees and employers is possible.

Workplace

A workplace is a designed social facility comprised of individuals who function toward the attainment of corporate goals; a workplace is a designated facility or area where work is performed. It may be an internal or external environment, it may have a structured organizational reporting system or it may be *laissez faire* in reporting relationships. Workplace policies, procedures and philosophy govern the organization's actions, and recognition of past precedence is a consideration in all DM activities. Workplaces provide an environment of unique physical and mental stressors. Ultimately, those with the most success have philosophies that support and recognize employee contribution as discussed in *Fortune* magazine's 1998 list of the top 100 companies to work for worldwide where it shows a clear link between job satisfaction and productivity (Robbin & Langton 2001).

It is known that organizational health and corporate culture have an influence on an employee's desire to stay at work or RTW following illness or injury. Yardley (2003) highlights the necessity of having a healthy organization to gain and maintain the results and wellbeing of the employees. Lack of a 'healthy workplace' philosophy and relationship can create an organization and/or individual susceptible to potential damaging interactions. In the model it is recognized and addressed that factors beyond the job itself have a significant influence on DM outcomes.

Clearly, company philosophy plays a part in DM outcomes. However, this is not meant to minimize the impact of the actual physical condition. It is essential that appropriate treatment and 'job fit' is considered in the model. Accurate and current job descriptions – which reflect the work and the required skills, capabilities and knowledge, as well as potential hazards and their control – will add to the ability to perform appropriate job matches. These will provide valuable information for the DM practitioner and those involved in the employees' treatment and care. The DM practitioner needs to be aware of the workplace physical risk factors in addition to the psychological factors and address these fully.

The importance of workplace endorsement and full organizational support are a necessity of the DM process.

A number of assumptions are built into the model including:

- The workplace is not self-contained: it interacts with providers, suppliers and customers.
- The workplace has physical attributes and risks.
- The workplace has many interactions with family, community and environment.
- Workplace attitudes can influence the outcome of disabilities.

Workers

Workers are central to the model and have physiological and psychological needs. The type of injury or illness, and the employee reaction to the condition, will have an influence on DM outcomes. The disabled worker is one individual in a workplace comprised of many individuals.

Workers can vary significantly in their conditions and motivations. There are different physical and psychological capabilities, personalities, fitness levels, wellbeing values, age, lifestyles, pre-existing conditions, and overall beliefs and values. Workers' responses to disability can be influenced by many individual variables in the inner and outer spheres of the model. Responses may also include a worker's internal psychological makeup, their beliefs about their locus of control and their inherent level of hostility or mistrust.

The collection of individual worker demographics and characteristics influence the design and implementation of a specific workplace DM programme. The domain focuses on the worker in the workplace but may be extended to embrace the comprehensive concept of the workplace community and interactions with the external community. A number of assumptions are used in this component of the model including that workers

- have lives outside of work that affect behaviours
- respond to injury and illness in very different manners
- are rational human beings capable of responsibility for their own actions.

Management

Management sets the philosophy and establishes the goals of the organization. These are reflected in the company mission and strategic plan and process and cascade to the operational level. Policies, procedures and processes evolve from the companies' goals, and objectives guide the operation of the business. In large corporations it should be recognized that local operating units may derive policies and procedures from those promulgated by the corporation but will ultimately implement them with a unique style. An underpinning of corporations is that they are in business to make profits, the relationship with employees is to exchange their time, expertise and effort for the execution of specific tasks. There are often competing needs with employers wanting to maximize efficiencies and employees exerting an amount of effort that they feel adequate and necessary to collect a pay cheque. This push-pull relationship needs to be considered in the DM programme design.

Organizational culture is an interesting influence and often provides stability to an organization's operating milieu. It gives employees a clear understanding of 'the way things are done around here'. Culture sets the tone for how organizations operate and how individuals within the organization interact.

The worker-and-management interactions – including the communication and reciprocal actions or influences between employees and management – often influence disability outcomes. Employee fit with the corporate culture is a variable in the DM process.

Imagine a situation where the CEO's executive administrator goes off on disability. Just prior to this there had been friction between the CEO and the administrator about turnaround time on projects, telephone manner and manager complaints on attitude. While off work, the executive administrator is replaced with an employee who has a high level of efficiency, a very positive disposition and a more intuitive response to the CEO's needs. Ultimately these circumstances will affect the CEO's desire to encourage the early return to work of the employee and create a complexity that will need to be dealt with in the DM process.

Management of human resource practices and policies defines the definite courses of action adopted by leadership in the organization. Consideration needs to be given to rotating leadership, fickle management strategies, inconsistent applications, short-term focus and continuous improvement initiatives. It has been clearly documented that employees are more likely to leave an organization due to poor management than they are the actual work (Duxbury et al 2003). Therefore, management attitudes to disability need to be understood and directed by corporate support for the DM efforts to succeed.

A number of assumptions about management are made with this component of the model: organizations have a desire to direct their managers to reduce the cost and consequences of disability, and organizations are clear in their strategic focus.

Co-workers

Interactions in the workplace can add an interesting dimension to the DM programme. Co-workers can be a point of interaction, and may offer support or become bullies depending on the acceptable behaviours in the workplace. In a situation where co-workers put unnecessary pressure on returning workers to 'pull their own weight' or work outside their restrictions the impact may be negative. On the other hand, co-workers who are supportive of workers (when transitioning back to work) can be a great asset to the DM programme. Additionally, co-workers may use their past experiences to project their reaction to the worker's disability.

Union

Unions have existed for more than 200 years and found a position in many workplaces. They feel they provide a collective voice for workers in workplaces. Workplaces with unions need to consider the role of the union and the concerns they have for their members who may encounter disabilities that are either work or non-work related. Unions, as with other types of organizations, are interested in helping disabled people and realize that they are a unique resource, which makes possible their special contribution to the workforce.

In working with unions a number of dimensions need to be considered: participation attitude; inherent biases against management suggestions or programmes; personal agendas (proximity to negotiations); rotating leadership; base knowledge level; and the local versus national perspective. Depending on dimensions, relationships, type of industry and location an employer may or may not have a joint labour management committee involved in the DM programme.

Assumptions

Unions have the best interests of their members as a value.

External factors

There are many external elements that can influence the DM process and outcomes. In this component of the model, the non-workplace influencers are defined as the context within which the worker lives and functions as a member of society outside the workplace. It is the world separate from the workplace, which, none the less, affects the work experience and worker responses to varying degrees.

Many elements can influence the climate in the external environment. The political and regulatory atmosphere that governs people's lives and their workplaces may have an influence. A striking contemporary example is the Ontario Workplace Safety and Insurance Board (WSIB) RTW efforts, which have driven dramatic changes in the likelihood of employers to re-employ following a workplace injury. As a positive example the current RTW legislation created an expectation that employers re-employ workers with work-related injuries. The legislation further stipulates that workers will participate in RTW efforts. This, combined with other initiatives, has resulted in a 20% decrease in the duration of claims over the past 10 years (WSIB 2002).

A social climate consists of a myriad of formal and informal human inter-relationships and circumstances among and within a human being's day-today functioning. Attitudes, beliefs, values, past experiences and proactive pursuit of health at any time can drive responses and interactions. Key external factors include family, advocates, social support, employee assistance programmes (EAPs), community agencies, culture, expectations, safety agencies, insurance or third-party administrator, workers' compensation, healthcare and lawyers.

Family

The family and the individual's role in the family can have an impact on the progression and outcome of the disability. If the individual is the primary 'bread winner' he or she may have a stronger desire to return to full duties faster to prevent wage loss. It has been proven that single mothers return to work faster than others with the same conditions. This is likely by virtue of the financial necessity and the contribution work makes to their lives. Alternatively, if the worker provides a second income in a family the inherent need to rejoin the workforce may not be as strong.

Advocates

Advocates often exist in the disability process; their influence could be negative or positive.

Social support

An individual's social support system may have an enabling or disabling effect. It is important to have such systems to provide a balance of positive reinforcement to become well and provide empathy. Social systems can also present problems with negative reinforcement when they provide secondary gain to support the disability status. As an example, a woman sustains a wrist injury and no longer has to do the laundry or the cooking. Her children join in and show tremendous concern for her health state. A great deal of pampering occurs and through no conscious decision the disability is prolonged. The secondary gain in this example is driving subconscious behaviour to remain disabled. The other side of this issue is the machismo that may exist in certain workplaces. As an example of this, each worker in a plant produces 500 parts per day. There is an unspoken productivity competition and the employees work beyond their physical capabilities to achieve higher production numbers. Even if their wrists ache, shoulders ache or other body parts start to break down, they do not mention it as that would be perceived as a weakness in that production environment.

Employee assistance programmes

Employee assistance programmes are often available to employees who want confidential interventions on psychological issues. These programmes may have a good short-term impact for non-complex situations. Critical thought needs to be exercised in designing these programmes so that the interventions escalate to a level that is required when necessary. EAPs do not generally deal with the issues that may be leading to or causing a disability. EAPs need to make sure they are using the right level of staff expertise to deal with complex psychological problems as, if this does not occur, it may create a situation where the issue is not dealt with in a manner that will resolve the root cause of the disability.

Community agencies

Community agencies may have a role to play within the model and offer valuable interventions depending on the level of disability. There are services such as assisted transportation and support groups that can be accessed when the disability warrants. Community services are often overlooked but available and could have an interaction with the worker's reaction to their disability.

Culture

Workforce diversity is highly valued and contributes positively to business outcomes. In disability situations it is important to recognize the implications of different cultural responses to disability. The need to respond to workers in recognition of these differences is essential. Some cultures may encourage more outward expression of pain where others encourage the individual to suffer silently. If positively managed by understanding and accepting the varying responses, attitudes and values can improve disability outcomes.

Expectations

Worker expectations can be formed by many elements, such as rumours, past experience, experience of others that they know, communicated process (e.g. employee brochures) and standard acceptable behaviours in the company. The interaction with the model is to realize that these expectations may exist and to deal with these as a method to resolve the issue and ultimately the disability. An example of this is, under the old Ontario Workers' Compensation System it was not uncommon to receive a disability pension for a relatively minor back injury. This meant that the worker went back to work with a 10% increase in wages. The worker right beside them doing the same task compared their income and status for performing the same work with the same physical exertion required. When the neighbouring worker experienced an injury they expected to receive a 10% increase in wages just like the other worker. This system no longer exists, but at the time it had a serious influence on expectations.

Safety agencies

The premise of many safety agencies is one of prevention and enforcement. In many workplaces this encompasses only work-related injuries or illness with little or no focus on personal health. Intervention by safety agencies may have an impact on the workplace depending on their involvement level. Safety agencies may have an impact on the interactions in the workplace. Particularly if the incident is considered 'critical' there will be a set of orders put to the employer to rectify the 'safety issue' that contributed to the incident. This intervention could have a positive effect on RTW if the changes were positive to the work environment, thereby making the job safer to perform.

Insurance and third-party administrator

There are many possible insurance or third-party claim administration possibilities. In workplaces that do have an organized system to adjudicate and manage short-term absences they may have an internal process, an external adjudication firm or an insurance company. The process is driven by adjudication and management of non-occupational claims. The method of adjudication and management of the claims at this third party can have an influence on outcomes. If a worker goes off work and the benefits are declined there are two possible outcomes:

1. The employee may return to work.
2. The employee may argue that the decision is incorrect and start to assemble more evidence that they are disabled. This could have negative consequences in that the employee will be focusing on supporting the claim instead of focusing on getting well. In assembling the supporting evidence for full disability the employee will begin to feel more disabled than originally diagnosed.

It is important for employers to select providers that handle denials in a positive RTW-focused manner and to guide the activities of external providers to support their internal DM strategies or early and safe RTW.

There are many workplaces that have no coverage for employees who are ill or injured non-occupationally. The availability (or lack of availability) of replacement income benefits can have an influence on the time off due to illness.

Workers' compensation

The interaction of the workers' compensation system can have an impact on the outcome of disabilities. The basic premise of the system is one of no-fault liability – if someone is injured at work they may receive compensation in the form of wage loss benefits, non-economic and/or economic loss awards, healthcare and rehabilitation assistance.

Some of the interactions that drive behaviours include the adjudication practices, claims management practices, RTW practices and appeal processes. The administration of claims through the various workers' compensation boards or insurers adds a complexity to the disability process. The system drives both employee and employer behaviours.

Healthcare

Healthcare availability and adequacy can have a significant impact on the outcome of disabilities. The interaction of healthcare within the comprehensive DM model is one of the greatest variables. In some disability cases, healthcare can create a systemic barrier to RTW and function. If the diagnosis is incorrect, if treatment is slow or inappropriate, or if services are inaccessible a profound detrimental effect can be seen. The impact on workers of substandard care is of longterm consequence.

The Romano Report (2002) highlights many of the challenges with the Canadian healthcare system and specifically identifies the lack of access of sometimes very needy individuals. This creates a negative influence on the DM process and, potentially, of prompt recovery.

Healthcare encompasses more than just physicians; it includes anyone who may be involved in the individual's care. Physical ailments may require physiotherapy or occupational therapy interventions. The philosophy of the treatment provider can have an impact on the eventual outcome of the treatment and success of the reintegration to the work.

Lawyers

If a lawyer becomes involved it can have an impact on the RTW and DM efforts. It may create a situation were the worker is arguing for benefits or higher permanent impairment ratings and gathering evidence to support the fact that they are disabled. A full understanding of the value (or lack of value) of legal interventions is not known but it is necessary to take this intervention and its financial impact into consideration when managing a claim.

CONCLUSION

Disability management practitioners need to adopt a model of practice that is appropriate for the health needs of their organization, for their corporate goals and for their corporate cultures. Disability management practitioners can use the conceptual model to understand the potential influences and identify the complex interactions at their worksites. Disability is not just about the ailment, it is influenced by the work, the workplace and external factors.

REFERENCES

Dooley D, Catalano R 1988 Recent research on the psychological effects of unemployment. Journal of Social Issues 44:1–12

Duxbury L, Higgins C, Coghill D 2003 Voices of Canadians: Seeking work-life balance. Conference Board of Canada Press, Ottawa

Feather N T, Bond M J 1983 Time structure and purposeful activity among employed and unemployed university graduates. Journal of Occupational Psychology 56:241–254

Frese M, Mohr G 1987 Prolonged unemployment and depression in older workers: a longitudinal study of intervening variables. Social Science Medicine 25:173–178

Goldenberg I, Goldenberg H 1980 Family Therapy: An overview. Brooks/Cole Publishing Company, Monterey, California, p 82

Heider F 1958 The Psychology of Interpersonal Relations. Wiley, New York

Jones E E, Davis K E 1991 Unemployment: the effects on social networks depression and reemployment opportunities. Journal of Social Science Research 15:1–22

Kelley H H 1967 Attributional theory in society psychology. In: Levine D (ed) Nebraska Symposium on Motivation. University of Nebraska Press, Lincoln, NE

Kielhoner G 1992 Conceptual Foundations of Occupational Therapy. F A Davis, Philadelphia, p 53

Pearlin L, Liberman M 1979 The social sources of emotional distress. Research in Community Mental Health 1:217–242

Riehl J P, Roy C 1980 Conceptual Models for Nursing Practice. Appleton Century Crofts, New York

Robbin S P, Langton N 2001 Organizational Behaviour: Concepts controversies applications. Pearson Education, Toronto, p 110

Romano Report (November 2002)
    www.hc.sc.gc.ca/english/pdf/romanow/pdfs/HCC_Final_Report.pdf

Tate R B, Yassi A, Cooper J 1999 Predictors of time loss after back injury in nurses. Spine 24(18):1930–1936

Winefield A H, Tiggemann M, Winefield H R 1991 The psychological impact of unemployment and unsatisfactory employment in young men and women: longitudinal and cross-sectional data. British Journal of Psychology 82:473–486

Winegardner D, Simmonetti J L, Nykodym N 1984 Unemployment: the living death? Journal of Employment Counseling 21:149–155

Workplace Safety and Insurance Board, Ontario 2002 Annual Report and Statistical Summary. www.wsib.org

Yardley J 2003 Three Critical Components for the Creation of Healthy Workplaces. Human Resources Professionals' Association of Ontario, p 43

Chapter 4

Disability management in the organization

LEARNING OBJECTIVES

- Understand the basic operations of an organization
- Identify how organizations plan
- Determine how to influence support in the organization
- Explore the formulation of goals and objectives
- Understand the need for cost–benefit analysis

INTRODUCTION

This chapter provides an overview of the basics on how organizations operate, possible structures, strategic planning, how to influence the organization internally and the essential elements of cost–benefit analysis planning. It is important to have an understanding of how organizations operate in order to gain and maintain support for overall disability management (DM) and return-to-work (RTW) programmes. The importance of senior management commitment for the DM programme is essential for the success of the initiative.

Almost everyone belongs to an organization, some may be small and some may be large. An organization can be a company, a not-for-profit endeavour, a self-help group or any configuration of a group of people who come together for a specific purpose. The ones that we will focus on are those that exist within an employment relationship. The majority of working-age individuals belong to an organization of this type. Some of the key features of organizations are that they are social entities, they have a structure, they are designed to achieve goals, they have distinct membership, they are relatively permanent, they use technology, they interact with their environments and they have structural dimensions (Das 1998).

Many of the key features of an organization are worth examining more closely when we consider the integration of DM into the corporation's operating realm. We recognize that organizations cannot survive without people to make the product or deliver the service, to make decisions about how, when and who will do what to ensure accomplishment of the goal. Corporations cannot exist without the human resources to accomplish their goals. Given this, organizations often have specific structures in place in a deliberate attempt to organize the workforce in a manner that can and will fulfil objectives by providing a method to direct, supervise and conduct the major activities.

BASICS OF ORGANIZATIONAL STRUCTURE

Organizations exhibit structural dimensions that need to be understood from the perspective of hierarchy, authority and distribution of task. All organizations have a structure under which they operate. This hierarchy denotes who reports to whom and for what, it delineates who the key decision-makers may be, it provides a framework for decision-making and it has been demonstrated (Druker 2002) that one of the most important variables in making any programme work in an organization is senior management's commitment and support.

There are many possible structures of an organization. However, the three most common are described as 'hierarchy', 'matrix' or 'flat' (Schermerhorn et al 1995):

■ *Hierarchy* This is the traditional structure with a clearly identified leader, whose title could be Chief Executive Officer (CEO) or President. The President then has key individuals reporting directly generally called Vice-Presidents. The Vice-Presidents then have a layer that reports to them and the hierarchy continues with directors, managers, lead hands and then the workers (Fig. 4.1).

Figure 4.1 The structure of a hierarchy.

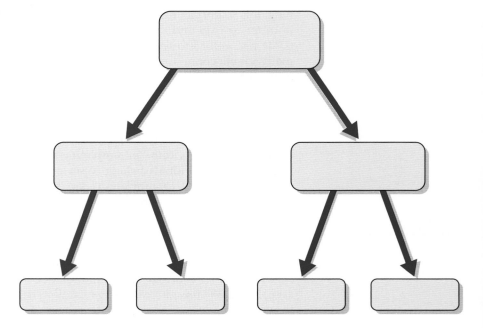

Figure 4.2 The structure of a matrix.

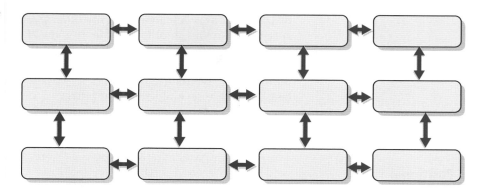

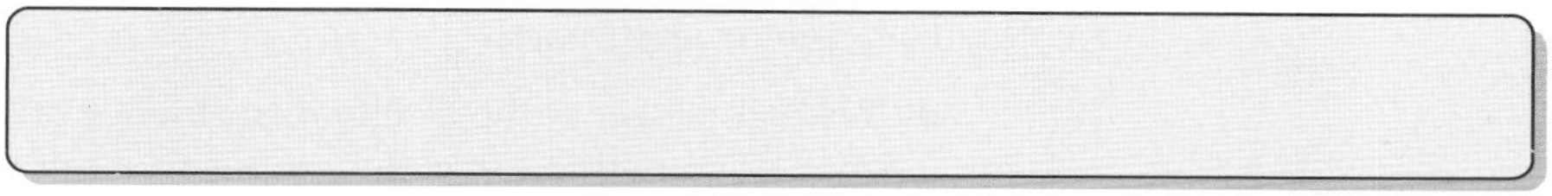

Figure 4.3 The structure of a flat organization.

- *Matrix* In this structure, departments interact closely with each other and although they still have departmental managers there is significant crossover between departments (Fig. 4.2).
- *Flat* This describes an organization with little, if any, authoritarian structure. This format is fairly common in entrepreneurial organizations (Fig. 4.3).

It is important to understand which type of organization you work within in order to ensure that you use the right channels to gain support for DM initiatives. The structure of the organization may be influenced by the business that the company participates in and the opinions of the ownership. A manufacturing environment may require a hierarchy in order to accomplish the production requirements in an efficient manner. Roles need to be defined and work allocated for performance. By comparison an information technology or sales organization may not require a structured reporting environment as most individuals will work independently and pursue personal targets. Size may also influence the type of structure; the smaller the organization the less likely the need for formal structure. It is important to recognize that in addition to the 'formal' organizational structure, informal arrangements, friendships and employee associations may influence the organization's operation.

EFFECTIVE LEADERSHIP

In corporations it is important for people to work collectively toward the accomplishment of the corporation's goals. It is an art to inspire people to perform necessary task to accomplish goals.

Dubrin and Harper (1997) define leadership as 'the key dynamic in the accomplishment of its objectives'. The foundations of effective leadership rest with the way a manager or any other person uses influence to obtain a specific behaviour in other people. It is the ability to make things happen. The organizational behaviour research on this topic discusses the use of power to influence actions. Good leaders use power in a positive manner to influence the willingness of others to work toward the accomplishment of task. There are several sources of power:

- *Positional* Reward; coercion; legitimacy
- *Personal* Expertise; reference.

Positional

Positional power would include managers and supervisors and is obtained due to an official status or position in an organization's hierarchy. In positional power there are three categories, which can be summarized as reward, coercion or legitimacy.

- Reward power is the ability to influence others through reward. It is the offer of something of value, a positive outcome as a means to influence the behaviour of others. This may include pay raises, promotions, special assignments, and verbal or written compliments.
- Coercive power is the ability to influence through punishment. The ability to punish or withhold positive outcomes as a means of influencing others. A manager may attempt to coerce someone by threatening them with verbal reprimands, penalties or termination.
- Legitimate power means influence through formal authority, the ability to influence behaviour through virtue of the rights of office or command, and the ability to act in the position of managerial responsibility.

Personal

Another source of power is the personal power that an individual can bring to a unique situation. This would be comprised of the personal qualities he or she brings. There are two main types of personal power.

- Expert power includes the ability to influence the behaviour of others because of one's specialized knowledge or understanding. Expertise derives from the possession of technical skills and know-how or information pertinent to the issue at hand, and which others do not have. This is developed by acquiring relevant skills or competencies, or by gaining a position where one's credibility displays one's true abilities.
- Referent power is the capability to influence the behaviour of others due to their desire to identify personally and positively with them. Referent power is power gained through charisma or interpersonal relations that encourage the admiration and respect of others.

Leadership is an important skill for DM practitioners in their roles within organizations. DM practitioners may be in situations where they will need to effect influence without a position of power within the formal hierarchy, thereby making leadership skills and an understanding of leadership in their organizations an important element of the job.

FUNCTIONS OF MANAGEMENT

Successful organizations recognize the value of a management process that enables the capability to plan, recognize problems and opportunities, make good decisions and take appropriate action. The functions of management can be summarized as four basic functions or responsibilities: planning; organizing; leading; and controlling (Schermerhorn et al 1995) (Fig. 4.4). They are defined as:

- *Planning* Setting objectives and deciding how to accomplish them.
- *Organizing* Arranging tasks, people and other resources to do the necessary work.
- *Leading* Inspiring people to work hard to perform according to plans.
- *Controlling* Monitoring performance and taking corrective action.

Planning

In order to define the direction and goals for the upcoming year organizations go through a strategic planning process. This will focus on key 'deliverables' which will assist in delivering the product or service and maintaining profitability. This process will identify the key focus areas that all employees will ultimately assist in achieving.

Figure 4.4 The management process.

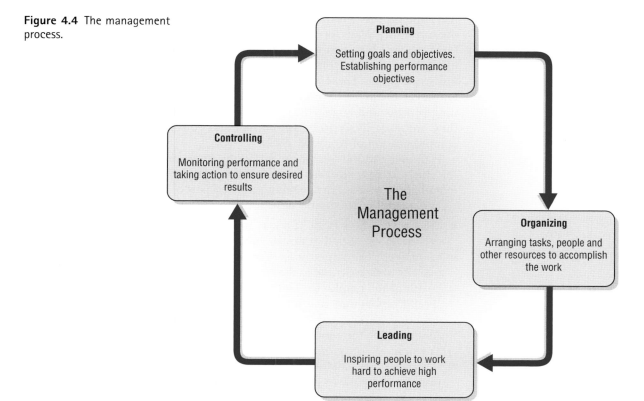

Strategic planning ensures a reasonable strategy and designs appropriate supporting structures to meet customer needs. Evolving from the strategic plan is a process of setting goals and objectives and deciding how to accomplish them. Organizations want to be sure that they have a plan outlining how they are going to achieve the desired outcomes. Planning can be formally defined as the process of setting goals and objectives and deciding how to accomplish them. Goals are broad statements quantifying the expected accomplishments and outcomes. Objectives are designed around the specific results that the organization wishes to achieve.

The planning process includes:

- setting/confirming the overall strategy and goal of the organization
- determining the current state
- developing an understanding about influencers on the future position, including a Strengths, Weaknesses, Opportunities and Threats (SWOT) analysis
- identifying and choosing appropriate objectives that will move the business forward
- implementing the action plan and evaluating results.

The importance of corporate planning cannot be underestimated as planning focuses attention on key strategic focus areas and places attention on key results.

The best type of strategic planning focuses the energies of the organization and cascades down through the various departments that need to establish strategic methods and objectives to fulfil their role in the delivery of the organization's plan. As discussed in Simmons (2002), if an employee senses inconsistency between what their bosses say and do it triggers a cascade of effects, depressing employees' trust, commitment and willingness to 'go the extra mile'. These effects reduce customer satisfaction and increase employee turnover, harming productivity. If managers are part of the planning process and engaged in the development of the goals and objectives they are more likely to be supportive and consistent in their pursuit and communication of company goals.

Planning and the establishment of objectives provides departments with the ability to measure results against these objectives. It also allows for correction if the results are not being achieved part of the way through the year.

The overall goals should have four key characteristics:

- *Measurable* There must be a way to reflect progress. 'What gets measured gets done.' Ensure that targets have a quantitative nature.
- *Meaningful* The target must represent something significant. The objective has to be essential to the success of resolving the disability and to the health of the employee. The worthiness of the goal must be apparent. It should be obvious that attainment of your objective will improve your employee's potential of returning to function and will increase the chances that the employer will have a valuable human resource back at work.
- *Achievable* The creation of an unreasonably aggressive goal serves no purpose. Actively or passively, participants will become discouraged and

drop out. The goal must be attainable in a realistic amount of time given current conditions and resources.

- *Challenging* Establish a goal that stretches the capabilities of the programme and the engagement of the absent employee. The objective must be realistic for those who will end up being participants. The ability to accomplish goals presents a positive impression on the programme.

Remember to be careful with the use of absolute goals such as 'no lost time' workdays or 'no longterm disability (LTD) claims'. While these are great ambitions and few would dispute the desire to have a world free of illness and injury, they represent an unrealistic future state. Establish significant but achievable goals.

Keep the employees in mind. Make sure you have a firm understanding of 'value' from their perspective even though this may not be as obvious as you think. Ensure that the attainment of goals will result in better service for the employee.

Establishing performance measurements and goals demands serious thought. It requires an understanding of the business operating vision and how the corporation views its employees.

Organizing

Organizing is the process of allocating resources and arranging the activities of individuals and groups to implement plans. Organizing turns plans into actions by defining tasks, assigning personnel and supporting them with technology and other material resources.

Leading

Leading is the process of arousing people's enthusiasm to support the organization's goals and to work hard to help accomplish important plans. Leading involves building commitments, encouraging work efforts that support goal attainment and influencing others to apply their best efforts on the organization's behalf. George and Brief (1992) assert that 'leaders who feel excited, enthusiastic and energetic themselves are likely to similarly energize their followers, as leaders who feel distressed and hostile are likely to negatively activate their followers'.

Controlling

Controlling is the process of monitoring work performance, comparing results to goals and taking corrective action as needed. This responsibility requires that managers follow work progress, that they maintain direct and active contact with people in the course of their work; and that they communicate regularly and on task-related concerns with the people doing the required work.

BUSINESS REASONS FOR MANAGING DISABILITY

A decrease in the human and financial costs of disability is frequently cited as a strong argument for the pursuit of DM initiatives (Bernacki & Tsai 2003, Kingery et al 2004, Loisel et al 2002).

A compelling argument for DM must focus on the positive impact DM can have on a company's bottom line and health outcomes for the employee. Green-McKenzie et al (2002) reviewed the implementation of a case management initiative that: included a specifically trained occupational health nurse case manager; included improved communication with treatment providers and employees; and included availability of transitional work. The results over a four-year period demonstrated a 20% decrease in claims, 46% decrease in lost time claims, and a 41% decrease in indemnity payments.

Absence, like turnover, can create significant costs for an organization. As discussed in Brown (2000) one *Fortune* 500 financial services corporation estimated the cost of absenteeism for 440 of their blue-collar and clerical workers at US$100 000.

Other studies have tied employee perceptions of the workplace to elements of productivity. The occurrence of psychological disability reflects the overall health of an organization. According to Perez and Wilkerson (1998), organizational health is an authentic employee health issue negatively influenced by 'excessive office politics, the failure to recognize honest effort, unclear job mandates, ambiguous direction setting by those in senior management, frequent changes in priorities and intrusive interruptions . . . lack of trust (and) poor communications'. Employers need to ask themselves what type of work environment they are promising then delivering to their employees.

Eisenberger et al (1990) found a positive relationship between employees' perceptions of being valued and cared about by their organizations and their attendance, dedication and job performance. Workers must feel secure about their status to fully engage themselves at work. This is a particular issue for low-status members of an organization, who cannot engage themselves deeply in their work when the organizational values do not fit their own.

Turnover is a significant and costly problem for many companies. The recruiting, staffing and training costs per person are estimated at US$5000 to US$10 000 for an hourly worker and between US$75 000 and US$211 000 for an executive at around the US$100 000 salary level. Auster (1998) estimates that replacement costs total 93% of the departing employee's annual salary. In addition, such a revolving-door situation means that employees are constantly moving along the learning curve instead of performing at full potential.

It is evident that employers need to address carefully how DM, just like training and development, effective leadership and attractive compensation, are part of creating a compelling and comprehensive employee value proposition that is founded on promises made to employees. Employers need to move beyond only looking at the traditional direct costs attached to disability. There is a need to recognize and address the bigger picture of the role that employee engagement, influenced by many factors including DM practices, has on corporate results. At the same time, employers need to understand the impact that workplace culture has on employee engagement, or in some cases the occurrence of disability (Curtis & Scott 2003).

As discussed in Amick et al (2000), 'work disability arises from complex interactions between the work environment and the individuals within it'. As Curtis and Scott (2003) state, 'sustaining a competitive advantage depends on optimizing valuable human resources'. Companies that are better able to recruit, develop and retain disabled employees will have an edge. Talented people will be attracted to corporations that value every employee's capabilities and will be more willing to invest themselves in productive activity if they believe they are treated fairly.

As discussed in Curtis and Scott (2004):

> Today's employers go to considerable lengths to attract talent by promising a position and work environment that is engaging and satisfying. Typically, this includes promises of development opportunities, attractive performance-based compensation, a commitment to employee wellness, empowered decision-making and effective leadership.

> When these promises break down, employees start to exhibit behaviours and symptoms that cost employers billions of dollars in turnover, lost productivity and illness/injury each year. Some employees may leave the company, some may stay and minimize their efforts and a fair number will travel down the unwanted road of disability.

> It is evident that employers need to carefully address how integrated DM, just like training and development, effective leadership and attractive compensation, is part of creating a compelling and comprehensive strategic initiative.

STRUCTURING THE BUSINESS CASE

Disability costs are substantive and in the big picture DM can contribute to a company's longterm financial performance and its short-term stock performance. However, the most successful business case for DM is one that focuses on contributing to the company's strategic plan and assisting in the attainment of its specific business objectives.

How the business case fits into the strategic and operational plan

It is important to include DM in the corporate strategic planning process. This means integrating DM as one component of the company's strategies to which its leaders are firmly committed. In doing so, the company clearly articulates the importance of effective human capital management, confirms its promises to employees and specifies which 'people processes' need to be in place to have a positive influence on business outcomes.

When effectively developed and implemented, DM addresses the reciprocal economic and humanistic needs of the two key stakeholders (the company and the employees) in organizational health. Successful workplaces are extremely rigorous in pursuing the key factors that shape health in the organization. This includes establishing and communicating performance measures in advance to determine the success of DM. The DM programme must clearly convey its objectives and measures to ensure that employees are engaged by the programme and are assisted back to wellness. This may require exploration of the underlying causes that affect employee engagement and can preclude an employee from returning to work (Curtis & Scott 2003).

Creating a business case for DM involves five steps:

1. Determining the fit with the strategic plan, business objectives and needs.
2. Conducting a gap analysis covering the present situation and the future desired state.
3. Identifying actions required for each objective or need.
4. Conducting a cost–benefit analysis.
5. Developing tracking mechanisms to assess progress and financial impact.

Determining the strategic plan fit and business objectives starts with consideration of the overall business strategy and identifies the highest-leverage business opportunities or needs that require DM interventions.

The second step is simply an analysis to identify the gap between where the company is right now and where it wants or needs to be in the future. 'How to' close the gaps becomes part of the goals and objectives of the DM programme.

The third step is identifying what is required to achieve these objectives or needs and deciding whether the nature and magnitude of the initiative will be focused or comprehensive in scope. A focused approach has targeted and specific objectives that seek a particular short-term payback of investment dollars. A comprehensive strategy has multiple targets and objectives.

The fourth step calls for identifying the costs involved in implementing the DM initiative compared to the expected returns/benefits. Return to investment is an important element in any corporate strategy.

The fifth and final step requires that a company identifies up front and along the way all the activities of progress that can be measured and evaluated. Building in such measures replicates the way most organizations assess business performance. It also reinforces the need for including measures and monitoring processes in strategic business plans that have timetables assigned accountability for rewarding and recognizing progress.

While many companies acknowledge the importance of making DM a *business* consideration, DM is often not a top *business* priority. Other *business* initiatives, which present more compelling hard (e.g. quantified) evidence of payback on investment, win out over DM initiatives, which seem to offer less predictable or quantified benefits. As a result, many DM practitioners revert to the argument that 'it's the right thing to do' and trust that management will back their suggestions to promote a DM philosophy, then wonder why nothing happens or why well-intended initiatives fail. The presentation of a solid *business case* increases the likelihood of obtaining the

Figure 4.5 The strategic fit. Align strategic plans for customers/employees and enabling tactics including leadership, employee development, empowerment, compensation/benefits and disability management. Strategic plans, customer value proposition, employee value proposition and enabling tactics interact horizontally and vertically to achieve performance targets. EBITDA: Earnings Before Interest, Taxes, Depreciation or Amortization. (Curtis & Scott, 2004)

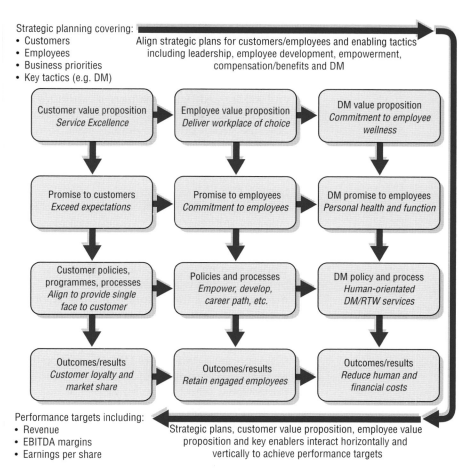

Strategic planning covering:
- Customers
- Employees
- Business priorities
- Key tactics (e.g. DM)

Align strategic plans for customers/employees and enabling tactics including leadership, employee development, empowerment, compensation/benefits and DM

Customer value proposition
Service Excellence

Employee value proposition
Deliver workplace of choice

DM value proposition
Commitment to employee wellness

Promise to customers
Exceed expectations

Promise to employees
Commitment to employees

DM promise to employees
Personal health and function

Customer policies, programmes, processes
Align to provide single face to customer

Policies and processes
Empower, develop, career path, etc.

DM policy and process
Human-orientated DM/RTW services

Outcomes/results
Customer loyalty and market share

Outcomes/results
Retain engaged employees

Outcomes/results
Reduce human and financial costs

Performance targets including:
- Revenue
- EBITDA margins
- Earnings per share

Strategic plans, customer value proposition, employee value proposition and key enablers interact horizontally and vertically to achieve performance targets

leadership commitment and resources needed to implement DM initiatives successfully.

Integration of DM into the corporate strategic planning process means integrating DM as one component of the company's human resource strategies to which its leaders are firmly committed. These strategies are then cascaded as corporate priorities, objectives and policies that become tactical programmes and processes at the activity planning level. In doing so, the company clearly articulates the importance of effective human capital or 'people' management, confirms its promises to employees and specifies which people processes need to be in place in order to influence employee engagement and business outcomes positively.

Figure 4.5 depicts how DM fits into comprehensive strategic planning. For illustrative purposes, the figure uses the example of a company that has decided to differentiate its customer value proposition by focusing on 'service excellence'. The depicted strategic planning model is equally available to companies with a different customer value proposition, such as product innovation or operational excellence.

Workplaces that meet the healthy organization and employee engagement challenges by integrating DM into strategic planning are well positioned to improve corporate results. Rucci et al (1998) note that one of the most notable examples of this relationship comes from Sears, Roebuck and Company. Through the 'Employee–Customer–Profit Chain', Sears identified and addressed how 'employee attitudes influenced customer service, employee turnover, and, ultimately, company profits'. This work illustrates how the vision of a 'compelling place to work' is linked through a series of outcome measures to strategic goals covering customer loyalty and profitability. In the end, the Sears model established the direct correlation between employee engagement and satisfaction, customer loyalty and bottom-line financial results.

The capacity of employees to deliver a company's customer value proposition is influenced by various workplace factors including DM efforts. Many variables influence the absence of disease, including the employees' perceptions of their health, and ability to function at work (Cole et al 2002). Understanding the disability experience as an organizational phenomenon, rather than simply a medical condition, leads to a broader consideration and management of the factors that directly or indirectly influence employee decisions on attending work and/or contributing to the company when at work.

Developing a *business case* for DM is more difficult than for other *business* issues because evidence of DM's impact on the bottom line has not been systematically measured and documented for easy retrieval and use. The DM professional who tries to build such a *case* confronts a vast array of information and advice, and can find little guidance on how to pull these data together to present a compelling and fact-based *business case from accessing business acumen.*

Just as the head of marketing must present a compelling, fact-based business case to top management to gain the necessary commitment and resources from the organization to pursue a product advertising launch, so too must the DM professional develop a case for DM integration based on the competitive edge gained by optimizing the people resources ('human capital') of the corporation.

CONVEYING THE IMPORTANCE TO SENIOR MANAGEMENT

From a company perspective, DM policies and programmes are intended to bridge personal and corporate health in order to achieve organizational objectives including enhancing employee engagement, reducing the human and financial costs of illness or injury, and enabling the company to achieve business objectives. This is why DM needs to be considered as a top business priority integrated into a company's strategic value and planning processes.

Setting goals

Much of the time management literature focuses on not just getting things done but on getting things done that are important to the organization.

Research indicates that people who set goals are more productive than those who do not. Some goal-setting ensures better results. There are a number of reasons why this is so. Goal-setting is an essential part of a larger activity, planning which involves:

- the identification of values, issues and problems
- goal selection
- choice of strategies
- decisions about operations and tactics
- monitoring
- assessment and revision of strategies and goals.

Goals are more obtainable if they are broken down into 'subgoals'. This brings task dimensions to goals and makes them appear manageable; bringing a structure to how goals will be achieved makes them seem more manageable. An effective process is to write down:

- long-term goals
- short-term goals
- for each short-term goal a number of subgoals
- monthly goals, which may be the same as the subgoals or result from a further breakdown
- weekly objectives that flow from each monthly goal.

To achieve weekly objectives a 'To Do' list can be used. It is even possible from a time-management perspective to block time on the calendar and log against these timeframes. Unfortunately, as we have all experienced, things always take longer than originally anticipated so estimate the amount of time required then multiply it by 1.5 to get a better sense of the time commitment. It is pointless to have monthly goals or weekly objectives that are not accomplished. The concept of a time log will also allow you to determine where time is being inefficiently spent and how this can be addressed if it is preventing the accomplishment of the task.

Deciding on priorities can also assist in focusing activity and increase the likelihood of completion. For example, a yearly goal might be able to identify those aspects that contribute to satisfaction with a RTW programme and those that contribute to dissatisfaction then develop strategies for increasing positive outcomes. A monthly goal may be to design an evaluation form that goes to the employee after the RTW to capture feedback adequately.

Monthly subgoals and weekly objectives should be based on measurable performance not outcomes. The reason for this is that often you will not have control over how you behave. For example, one monthly goal might be 'convene a meeting of the DM committee to review draft policy'. Contrast this with the goal of 'gain approval for draft policy' which you cannot ensure because it requires other people's cooperation. On the other hand, 'Develop a DM policy and provide information to employees on the policy and programme' may be an appropriate yearly goal.

- Goals and objectives should be precise, measurable and have deadlines. Vague goals may be difficult to break down and use in planning, and they are often not motivating because there is no clear finishing point that can be identified and enjoyed.

■ Goals should be realistic – not too difficult to obtain and requiring some stretch to improvement. Incremental changes in the short term can bring about enormous improvements in the long term.

■ Goals and objectives should always be stated in positive terms, e.g. what will be done rather than what will not be done.

■ Structuring goals, objectives and a plan to get there will increase the likelihood of achievement and ultimately the overall success of the programme.

Cost–benefit of RTW

It is important to measure the success of the DM and RTW initiatives to ensure company support for the programme. A baseline of information is a good starting point for overall cost–benefit analysis. Formulating the business case by use of a solid cost–benefit analysis is useful in gaining initial and ongoing corporate support.

Baseline data

Data can be collected from many sources in the organization. A number of departments may contribute to the information required for compiling these data including Human Resources, Finance and Payroll. External agencies may also be good sources of information including workers' compensation agencies, insurance companies or external third-party administrators/consultants.

Essential baseline data may include:

■ Overall workers' compensation costs, sick time, short-term disability, LTD and other absences.

■ *Workers' compensation data* Each workers' compensation board or insurer maintains employer data on cost, claims and trends. When analysing the workers' compensation costs remember to take into consideration the base premium plus any surcharge that may be allocated based on experience.

■ *Sick leave/Short-term disability* Employers may have employee sick-leave plans managed in-house or through a third-party administrator or a short-term disability insurance plan. If the employer does not have such plans employees who are ill may be able to apply for government disability benefits. Even though these are either funded by the company directly or jointly by employees and employers through payroll taxes or deductions, they should be counted from the loss of productivity standpoint. The information on these costs may be available from the payroll or finance department in the organization.

■ *Long-term disability* Some employers have LTD plans, which they self-fund or pay premiums for to an insurance company. There are many funding mechanisms for LTD benefits. However, the claim costs are an important consideration to include in the baseline data.

- *Other absences* Employers may have other types of absences and allowances for employees, such as family leave. It is worthwhile determining how many days are lost per year on these absences. Although employers may not be able to influence these lost days they can complete the absence picture of an organization.
- *Other data* Other programme data that may be of interest are the Employee Assistance Program data, drug plan data and extended health-benefit data such as the utilization of psychological services. These data would be available in aggregate from the third-party provider or insurer.

Internal baseline data

Internal baseline data should be available either in the DM department or from Human Resources, Payroll or Finance. The important categories, at a minimum, would include:

- number of lost days by benefits category
- costs of lost days per benefit category.

The data can be broken down further into the following categories:

- reason for absence and type of disability
- department
- job category
- supervisor
- age
- gender
- years of service.

Some employers will not have information about absences until there is a disability. Nevertheless, they can often find some absence information on their payroll systems. To dig out the information about employee absences, experts say employers have to make a concerted effort to track the data, starting with facts they might already have.

There are also many indirect costs. A lot of payroll systems collect overtime information. Frequently, overtime or replacements are needed to cover someone who called in sick or was out on disability. Estimates can be based on that information. Some employers can also review the time and attendance modules within their human resources information systems, while others could use timekeeping systems to detect absences associated with workers' compensation, sick time or unpaid leave.

It can be very difficult to capture all of the data if they are not being tracked or if they are not on paper or systems cannot communicate with one another. Still, employers can take an incremental approach: start with what you have and establish a baseline to understand current costs establishing parameters for data gathering and reporting mechanisms.

Some employers may also wish to do external benchmarking. The need for external benchmarks depends on corporate goals, and if one of your requirements within your business is to have a cost factor the same as your competitors, then you need to do this. On the other hand, employers who just want to control costs as much as possible do not necessarily need to benchmark.

Budgeting

One of the essential components of establishing a business strategy for claims is defining the budget. The information used in forming the appropriate goals and objectives will assist in establishing an adequate supporting budget.

Disability management and RTW budget processes will include estimates of what may be required in time, services, equipment and training. Once the budget has been established tracking is important since this information is required to evaluate the effectiveness of the DM programme.

Organizations will differ in which cost items they track. Some organizations do not include costs that they consider part of operating the business; others may include all costs. Some of the types of cost items that may be included in DM budgets are:

- sick leave or short-term disability payment cost
- disability insurance premiums
- workers' compensation premiums
- salary and benefits
- third-party services: third-party administrator, functional ability evaluations, independent medical examinations, physiotherapy and other assessments
- assistive devices/technology
- hardware and software
- other equipment and supplies
- communication costs, e.g. telephone and email
- education information costs, e.g. developing information for supervisors, employees and service providers
- professional development, e.g. journals, conferences and updating
- infrastructure costs, i.e. costs involved in providing space, accounting, upper-level management and supervision, legal support, etc.
- changes or renovations to the work environment or workstation
- rehabilitation: on-the-job training or retraining
- supervisor time, and time of other staff members
- other.

Benefits

It is very important to keep track of the savings or benefits realized as a result of the programme. These may include decreases in:

- premiums
- duration of lost time claims
- overtime
- replacement costs
- impact on employees.

Measures of success can be both quantitative and qualitative. The quantitative business measures demonstrate the decrease in hard dollar costs and accomplishments against goals and objectives. The qualitative results can be process measures. These can be evaluated by involving employees in focus groups, surveys, interviews and various audits or needs assessments. Process indicators enable top management to see signs of progress, even when business results are not yet visible.

Outcome measures provide validation and ultimate justification for the support and investment in DM. These include measures produced by initiatives designed to achieve specific business objectives, such as number of total lost time claims (LTCs), percentage of LTCs, cost of LTCs, number of days on transitional work, average cost per claim, overall costs, percentage of employees who successfully RTW, long-term disability rates and successful rehabilitation.

It is important to track the actual costs versus the benefits on a regular basis. If interim adjustments are required a cost–benefit analysis may allow for these variances. The benefits of bringing a disabled worker back to work are considerable.

In presenting the results of the business case for a comprehensive approach to DM, process measures should be communicated. Progress of the DM interventions, and outcome measures, which track the impact of DM on business results, need to be defined then results communicated regularly.

Communicating overall results

Communication is essential in the DM process. 'Communication is an interpersonal process of sending and receiving symbols with messages attached to them. This process is a foundation of all interpersonal relationships. Through communication people exchange and share information with one another; through communication people influence others' attitudes and behaviours' (Schermerhorn et al 1995).

Communication can be used to inform, influence, control, inspire and gain support. It is used all the way through the DM and RTW processes. An important time for communication is when conveying the results of the DM and RTW initiatives. In the organizational context, knowledge of how the organization operates will assist with the design of communication materials. If the organization is hierarchical the best approach may be a formal report or presentation. If the organization is informal a memo format may be the optimal communication medium. The most essential detail is that results are communicated to all key parties.

CONCLUSION

The bottom-line focus of today's business environment requires that DM initiatives be treated like any other important business strategy. Thus, DM professionals must create a clear, compelling business case linked to the company's strategic business objectives. By providing top management with a better understanding of the expected return on investment, DM practitioners can more successfully compete for the company's scarce resources, resulting in better-funded and -supported DM initiatives.

REFERENCES

Amick B C, Habeck R V, Hunt A et al 2000 Measuring the impact of organizational behaviours on work disability prevention and management. Journal of Occupational Rehabilitation 10(1):21–38

Auster E R 1998 Behind closed doors: sex bias at professional and managerial levels. Employee Responsibilities and Rights Journal 1:129–144

Bernacki E J, Tsai S P 2003 Ten years' experience using an integrated workers' compensation management system to control workers' compensation costs. Journal of Occupational and Environmental Medicine 45(5):508–516

Brown J 2000 Employee turnover costs billions annually. Computing Canada, December, p 25

Cole D, Mondloch M, Hogg-Johnson S for the Early Claimant Cohort Prognostic Modelling Group 2002 Listening to injured workers: how recovery expectations predict outcomes – a prospective study. Canadian Medical Association Journal 166(6):749–754

Curtis J, Scott L 2003 Making the connection. Benefits Canada, April:75–79

Curtis J, Scott L 2004 Integrating disability management into strategic plans: creating healthy organizations. American Association of Occupational Health Nurses Journal 52(7):298–301

Das H 1998 Strategic Organizational Design. Prentice Hall, Scarborough, Ontario

Druker P 2002 Managing in the Next Society. St Martin's Press, New York

Dubrin A J, Harper A 1997 Essentials of Management, 4th edn. ITP Nelson, Toronto

Eisenberger R, Fasolo P, Davis-LaMastro V 1990 Perceived organizational support and employee diligence, commitment, and innovation. Journal of Applied Psychology 75(1):51–59

George J M, Brief A P 1992 Feeling good – doing good: a conceptual analysis of the mood at work–organizational spontaneity relationship. Psychological Bulletin 112(2):310–329

Green-McKenzie J, Rainer S, Behrman A et al 2002 The effect of health care management initiatives on reducing Workers' Compensation costs. The Journal of Occupational and Environmental Medicine 44(12):1100–1105

Kingery P M, Ellsworth C G, Corbett B S et al 2004 High cost analysis: a closer look at the case for worksite health promotion. Journal of Occupational Medicine 36:1341–1347

Loisel P, Lemaire J, Poitras S et al 2002 Cost-benefit and cost-effectiveness analysis of a disability prevention model for back pain management : a six-year follow-up study. Occupational and Environmental Medicine 59:807–815

Perez E, Wilkerson B 1998 Mindsets. Mental Health – The ultimate productivity weapon. Homewood Centre for Organizational Health, Guelph, Ontario

Rucci A J, Kirn S P, Quinn R T 1998 The employee–customer–profit chain at Sears. Harvard Business Review on Point, Jan–Feb:83–97

Schermerhorn J R, Catteneo R, Templer A 1995 Management: The competitive advantage, 2nd edn. John Wiley, Toronto

Simmons T 2002 The high cost of lost trust. Harvard Business Review, September:18–20

Chapter 5

Disability management and prevention

INTRODUCTION

Prevention of disability is a broad topic which can encompass everything from corporate culture, through health and safety, ergonomics, engineering design, accident investigation, root cause analysis, employee selection, to health promotion programming. As part of disability management (DM) programme planning it is necessary to look at each workplace as unique and decide whether risk exists and how to address it to decrease the prevalence of disability. It would be impossible to give each of these topics a full review so we have broken them down into corporate culture, health and safety, and health promotion to provide a high-level summary of the types of intervention that have a significant impact on preventing the disability from occurring.

It is important when looking at DM that areas of culture, health and safety, and health promotion be examined. Disability is a complex combination of contributing factors. 'Recent evidence has demonstrated that disability from musculoskeletal disorders is a multifactor problem due to the causal disorder, workers' global characteristics (physical and mental), and environmental factors, such as the workplace, the health-care system, the compensation system, and the interactions between all stakeholders in the disability problem. This evidence suggests that the typical disease-focused treatment paradigm should be replaced by a disability prevention paradigm to avoid long term disability' (Durand et al 2002).

The characteristics of an organization and its employees are an important variable in planning any DM management prevention strategy. Figure 5.1

Figure 5.1 The intertwining of disability prevention into the overall strategy.

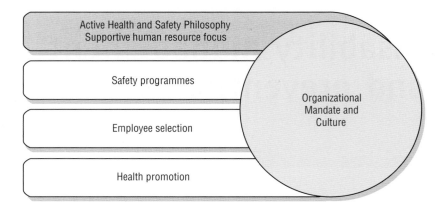

demonstrates the intertwining of disability prevention into the overall strategy.

CORPORATE CULTURE

Management makes a conscious decision about accepted behaviours and policies surrounding their business operation and human resources. Organizations exist for specific purposes; they hire people that will help them advance that purpose and value those that assist in the accomplishment of their goals. An organization's culture is reflected in its strategic and operational plans and the importance of the human element in the plans' execution. However, the human relationship is a complex combination of skills, capabilities, knowledge and emotions. Each individual is different and will respond to situations differently based on inherent intellectual, physical and emotional capability, past experiences and current circumstances.

Even with the right overall corporate culture, aberrations can occur due to individual circumstances. For example, an individual could be a high-functioning member of a team in one circumstance, but transition to a new circumstance and due to group dynamics, poor management support, alternate corporate culture or other variables is regarded as a low contributor. McCall (1998) discusses how individuals can become targets of poor management behaviours, and career destruction results. In some cases the individual will move on to challenges that are better suited to them, in others they may end up on disability. Imagine a case where a man was a high-performing supervisor with terrific results so the corporation promoted him to become a manager at another site. The product was the same, the environment was similar and he successfully turned production output in a positive direction by implementing standards and processes that existed in the workplace where he had accumulated his experience and knowledge. Imagine the same man being promoted into an environment with a different circumstance. For example, he is promoted into the position and used the same strategy as above. However, one of the supervisors who now reported to him had also been up for the promotion but lacked the capability or results to obtain the promotion. Unfortunately, bitterness drove the supervisor to undermine all of the new manager's initiatives and to try to sway other team members into not supporting the new initiatives. Add to the equation that the director who had facilitated the promotion was moved to an alternative area of responsibility, taking away any potential balance to the negative interventions by the angry supervisor. Then include that the replacement for the director who had facilitated the promotion was weak, inexperienced and had a pre-existing close personal relationship with the supervisor who did not get the promotion. Suddenly, a very successful manager with proven knowledge and skills is of no importance and in fact being 'beaten up' by the corporation due to personal factors beyond his control. The outcomes are bound to be very different. One potential outcome is that the manager transitions to disability due to ongoing psychological abuse by the director and the direct supervisor report. Although this scenario does not reflect the entire culture of the corporation, if the corporation allows these behaviours to occur it creates an inconsistency that employees will notice. Relationships and interactions are not simple, and corporations need to recognize that there are many influences on disability. Consistency in application of corporate culture is essential. As discussed in Kirsh (1996) one of the most important elements in solid working relationships is trust. Employees need the security of knowing how the corporation will respond in a given situation and the consistency of a supervisor's decisions and responses.

The prevention of disability is a complex web of interactions. It is essential to build crosschecks into the system to ensure that consistent messages are delivered and that issues such as the above case can be resolved prior to the disability outcome.

An example of how corporate culture influences outcomes can be found in mergers and acquisitions situations. There are many unknowns in these situations and the organization that has a culture of keeping employees informed will reduce the amount of anxiety and uncertainty involved in stressful transitions. If employees are unaware of what future they hold with the organization they may decide to explore avenues of securing their income levels including disability benefits. The data clearly demonstrate an increase in the number of claims prior to lay-offs or directly following mergers and acquisitions due to the potential threat of job loss. If the organization spent sufficient time communicating with employees about direction and the future state the incidence of disability could be reduced.

As discussed in the Michigan Disability Prevention Study (1993), corporate culture can be reflected in positive work relationships with employees, positive morale, attention to interpersonal skills, open communication, regular and meaningful involvement of employees in company operations, and decisions and sharing and seeking of information. It is important that corporations not only define their culture but live by those definitions.

HEALTH AND SAFETY

Safety practices, policies and procedures – which are integrated directly into the standard operating procedures, safety expectations and goals, and built into supervisor performance appraisals – have a high potential for driving safety success.

Positive health and safety programming encompasses:

- corporate culture
- senior management support
- union support (if applicable)
- accountability at all levels of the organization
- worksite hazard identification and correction processes
- prevention programmes, including appropriate engineering design, ergonomic considerations, preventative maintenance, housekeeping, standardized safe work practices and training
- corrective action
- accident investigation and root-cause analysis
- emphasis on safety and safe behaviours
- personal history.

Safety must be a central part of work operations; safe behaviours need to be endorsed as the normal expectation.

Corporate culture

An example of the influence of corporate culture is tolerance for risk-taking behaviours. In a work environment there should be zero tolerance for unsafe acts. However, most of us can think of at least one example that we have seen where an individual has taken a short cut and it has become an accepted behaviour. Construction is one of the professions with a high risk of short-cut behaviour because it may be perceived as faster not to secure an object, or not to shore a trench. If the supervisors do not embrace a safety philosophy and reinforce the fact that not shoring the trench is an unacceptable risk behaviour it can have serious consequences for the workers. Safe behaviours must be reinforced and at times enforced to ensure they occur. Tolerance for unsafe behaviour is clearly something worked into the cultural fabric of the organization.

Although health and safety is predominantly associated with work-related injuries and illness many of the lessons will overflow into an employee's personal life. The direct impact of quality health and safety programmes is clear in reduced workers' compensation claims. Health and safety programmes require detailed guidelines for the operation of equipment, production processes and the overall facility. This requires a positive atmosphere of safety, where employees are aware that an expectation of the job is to perform it safely.

Workplace hazard identification

Many considerations exist in the area of safety interventions including the type of job, workforce characteristics and availability of experts. The types of jobs being performed at the worksite are very important from a disability prevention point of view; in its simplest terms, white-collar bank employees do not have the same needs as those working in a manufacturing press shop. Therefore, one of the first important elements is recognition of hazards and design of prevention programmes geared to these risks. Safety is often common sense put into action. A taxi based in the inner city may need to consider shatterproof glass between the driver and the passenger, an emergency notification system, a cash-control system and other seemingly obvious safety precautions. However, a taxi based in a small farming community may not require such elaborate safety and security devices.

Prevention programmes

Health and safety orientation and ongoing training is of importance in all workplaces; workforce characteristics can guide prevention programmes to a great extent. If you have a workplace that is predominantly highly educated it is much different from a work environment where semiskilled employees are working on the factory floor. Some of the important characteristics when designing disability prevention programmes are age, gender, marital status, level of education, work history and job titles, accident history and nationality/language background. The work and the current distribution of accidents will assist in guiding interventions. The combination of data and employee information can help gear the interventions and potential programmes.

It is important in the safety area to adequately mention the design of equipment and production process areas. The science of safety and ergonomics has advanced to new levels. However, it has been slow to enter the engineering curriculum or undergraduate classroom. Ultimately, equipment is still designed that does not meet the needs of the employees who operate it. An example that comes to mind is a blow moulding press observed in a workplace that required the employee to reach overhead 20 times an hour to twist a knob. There was no legitimate production reason as to why the knob could not be at waist height. This is an example of poor design that will ultimately result in injury. Another prevalent design flaw is the height of conveyor belts, even though the average height of society has increased, conveyor belts are still designed for people 5 feet 7 inches tall (1.7 m), making the line too low for the majority of the workforce in North America, again creating a health and safety risk that may result in accidents and injuries. It is possible to design out many of the risk factors that exist in work environments.

Another important element in safety programmes is preventative maintenance. Equipment requires preventative care in order to ensure it continues to function to production and safety standards. Many maintenance departments have scheduled maintenance of the equipment based on manufacturers' guidelines. It is essential to make sure these are complied with and that any repair issues are immediately addressed. Excellence in preventative maintenance and equipment maintenance is of direct importance.

Safety training should be provided for all employees upon orientation, then periodically reinforced by supervisors and managers as an important job element. Compliance with safety rules and regulations is also a necessity in the prevention of work-related incidents. If an accident occurs it is essential that it is given sufficient attention with a prompt investigation and immediate action to resolve the safety hazard. It is not sufficient to find the obvious reasons for accidents – root-cause analysis must be performed. If an employee has a chemical splashed in his or her eye the obvious cause would be that the employee was not wearing personal protective equipment. However, if we look deeper into the root cause it might be found that the chemical drum was not labelled or the employee was new in the plant or the personal protective equipment was not available. It is apparent that there are many fixes to prevent this incident from occurring again once the root-cause analysis is performed. The attention to accidents needs to be not only at the plant-floor level but also at the senior-management level. Accident details and action plans to prevent future occurrences need to be reviewed at management meetings with the same importance as production scheduling and demands.

Another clear factor in accident behaviours and ultimately prevention is the attention that is given to accidents when they do occur. In workplaces that try to determine the root cause and fix it the number of incidents is significantly reduced. This is amplified in workplaces that not only perform root-cause analysis but include health and safety results in senior management meetings and performance appraisals. Accountability for safety results will drive safety behaviour.

Pre-existing conditions and post-offer screening

A worker's individual history is an interesting topic to explore given that it creates situations where the individual may have some pre-existing propensity to injury or re-injury due to personal conditions or residual symptoms or 'weakness'. Many employers, as part of their hiring process, will include a post-offer screen to determine if the candidate has the inherent capabilities to perform the job. The overall objective of post-offer screening is to protect the worker from harm and the employer from needless costs associated with that harm. Employing workers who meet objective job standards will result in reduced incidence and reduced severity of work-related musculoskeletal illnesses and injuries (Scott 2003). A study conducted by Chaffin et al (1978) clearly indicated that back injuries are more severe and return to work is delayed, and that the mean incidence and severity rates increase at a ratio of about 3:1, when the physical requirements of the job are more demanding than the workers' abilities.

As Hogan and Arneson (1991) discussed, the employee needs to be physically capable of performing the work or accidents can result due to a simple inability to perform that work. Therefore, one of the best ways to reduce costs due to injuries is to select individuals who are physically qualified to perform the work. In Nassau (1999) it was found that the severity of back sprains or strains, related medical costs and lost workdays were significantly lower with the use of pre-work functional screenings of all new employees hired for physically laborious jobs.

Effective post-offer screening programmes compare the employee's capabilities with the essential job requirements. Fleishman (1979) encouraged the use of fair screening procedures to ensure appropriate job selection. It is necessary to use proper job analysis techniques to determine the demands of the job and the relevant worker abilities. According to Fleishman, 'There is no such thing as general physical proficiency', the actual performance criteria need to be developed based on job demands not overall physical fitness.

The disability prevention case for the implementation of post-offer screenings is compelling.

Description of post-offer screening

Post-offer screening is a valid and reliable tool for identifying candidates' physical capabilities compared to the essential physical demands of the job, i.e. the outcome of post-offer screening is to determine if there is a match between the individual's functional capabilities and the physical requirements of the job. A comprehensive post-offer screening will include a physical demands analysis, clear acceptable criteria, standardized objective test, and occupational and job specific test.

Physical demands analysis

A physical demands analysis (PDA) involves a detailed examination of a particular job and the individual tasks associated with that job. A thorough PDA will include as much detail as possible including weights, forces, frequency, duration and pictures of all tasks performed. The PDA is the foundation of an accurate post-offer screening programme as it is used to match the applicant's abilities to a specific set of job demands.

Clear acceptable criteria

It is important to design acceptance criteria to ensure that the employer and the testing facility are clear about the testing parameters. All potential candidates must go through the screening process; job placement is conditional on meeting the physical requirements of the job. The facility performing the test must have a clear understanding of the minimally acceptable criteria as they relate to the essential physical demands of the job. This ensures that all candidates are measured against the same standardized criteria. For example, if the criterion is to lift 10 lb (4.5 kg) from the floor, it is important to measure the capability to perform this lift based on the requirement. 'Where cut off scores are used, they should normally be set so as to be reasonable and consistent with normal expectations of acceptable proficiency', according to Biddle and Nikki (1999). This component of planning requires some thoughtful analysis because it must withstand the rigour of discussion and challenge if a candidate is found unable to perform the work. The value of policies and procedures for the post-offer programme cannot be understated. Policies and procedures should specify the components of the programme, including goals, objectives and process to ensure consistency and success (Scott 2003).

Standardized objective test

Health professionals perform a musculoskeletal examination, including questions related to the individual's health and health history. The objective evaluation includes spinal and extremity range of motion, strength testing, and neurological examination of the upper and lower extremity reflexes, sensation and coordination. Specific tests to rule out the most common injuries seen in the prospective job are also included. The evaluator performing the objective computerized functional testing is able to reach a reliable conclusion related to the appropriateness of the applicant to meet the requirements of the job.

Computerized objective tools are available to assist evaluators with post-offer screening. Prospective employees complete a series of objective computerized tests (relevant to the demands of the job) creating an accurate measure of current capabilities. 'Functional testing can demonstrate an individual's level of safe physical performance and better direct the potential employee to a task for which he or she is suited', according to Randolph (2000).

Using a computerized tool has several advantages over testing an individual's function manually. First, the computerized tool automatically collects objective data, thereby removing any evaluator variance, and allows the evaluator to observe the actions and body mechanics of the prospective employee. Second, a large normative database allows the evaluator to compare the applicant's results to industrial norms. Therefore, the applicant is classified not only in terms of strength level but also with respect to the specific physical demands of the job. Third, a standardized objective test is a reliable tool that has credibility in a court challenge (Dakos & Scott 2001).

Occupational and job-specific testing

Occupational testing simulates functional parameters such as carrying, lifting, reaching, walking, sitting, standing, bending, twisting, kneeling, crouching, climbing and other activities integral to the applicant's work-related activities, i.e. the testing replicates specific job demands. For example, when testing for lifting capacity, if the worker must lift in confined spaces or walk around with the object, it is important to test for these job-specific demands. Simulating these components provides the evaluator with an insight into how the applicant would perform these tasks on site.

According to Randolph (2000), 'Functional capacity evaluation now stands in some jurisdiction as a mainstay of safe job placement and risk diminution by providing objective data pertaining to an individual's ability to safely perform job tasks'.

Case study

In a study conducted by Scott (2003) at a large, multinational, industrial employer to determine if post-offer screening reduced the number of injuries and the resulting costs post-hire it was proven that the post-offer screening was a valuable prevention tool. The data for the study were gathered throughout the hiring process and tracked for four years. The objective of the study was to determine whether or not the implementation of post-offer screenings would be a cost-effective initiative to implement company-wide and to determine whether post-offer screening could reduce the number of injuries and resultant suffering. The study used the process outlined above.

A group of 220 new hires participated in the study, 110 participated in post-offer screening and 110 did not. No other differences were found in the hiring practices or the post-hire work to be performed. The group of employees ($n = 110$) who had been screened post-offer were compared to a group of employees ($n = 110$) who had not been screened, then tracked for post-hire injuries and the resultant costs. Age, gender, ethnicity and pre-hire disability status were also tracked and, using chi-square analysis, no differences were found between the two groups on these variables of interest ($P < 0.05$).

Of the screened group, 92 (83%) passed the post-offer screening and 18 (16%) did not. Only those passing the screening were placed in the jobs offered. Individuals who did not meet the physical requirements could retest for alternative jobs and potentially become employed in a position consistent with their functional capabilities. The control group was not screened, so all the employees were placed in the jobs that had been offered.

A substantial difference was found between the groups in relation to the number of injuries sustained and the resulting post-hire costs (Table 5.1). The group that had post-offer screenings and, therefore, were known to have the physical capabilities to perform the jobs had only a 1% injury rate during the four years. The group that did not have post-offer screenings experienced a 23% injury rate during the four years: a substantial difference in injury rates between the two groups. Additionally, the cost of injuries for the screened group was much less than those in the non-screened group. In this case, post-offer screening clearly impacted positively on the number of occupational injuries and their resultant costs (Scott 2003).

The findings of this case study are important to employers, employees and DM practitioners. Clearly, the findings support the development of post-offer screening programmes as a disability prevention tool.

Table 5.1 Injuries and costs in group 1 and group 2[a]

	Injured employees	Non-injured employees	Injury costs (US$)
Group 1 (screened)	1	91	6500
Group 2 (not screened)	23	87	2 073 000

a Group 1: $n = 110–118$ employees who did not pass the screening; group 2: $n = 110$

PERSONAL CHARACTERISTICS

Employees may have previous personal experiences with disability, injury or illness that do not prevent them from performing the job but do create situations where the employee may reference their past experience and anticipate the same or similar outcomes. If they had a negative experience it may, in fact, have a negative influence on their response to a new injury.

This would also be true if they had a close friend or family member who had experience in the system, again referring to their good or bad experiences to judge the potential outcomes and responses. This brings us back to the discussion of capability to perform the assigned job. As discussed in Gilliam (2004), 'Rates of disability are on the rise fueled by a growing obesity epidemic. Individuals are less physically fit and this impacts on their ability to perform physically demanding jobs. Over 60 percent of the American workforce is either overweight or obese'.

HEALTH PROMOTION

Many health promotion programmes exist which can be introduced into workplaces. As discussed in Balch (2002), research demonstrates that approximately half of all illnesses are preventable with lifestyle changes and physical activity. The positive benefits of having a captive audience in the workplace can assist with changing health behaviours. However, it is important to understand the work group's needs prior to implementing these programmes. If there are no smokers in the work group a smoking cessation programme will, of course, be of little value. Data and demographics can be analysed to establish the priority needs of the work groups. Additionally, it is important to gear health promotion programmes not just to the data but to employee interest. Packaged health promotion programmes are of little value unless they look at the needs of the workplace. The most important variable in changing lifestyle behaviours is that the individual has to see a reason to change and want to change. There are many resources available when designing health promotion programming to address workplace needs.

Adult learning principles play an important role in the delivery of health-promotion programmes – gearing the message to the audience is as important as the message itself. A well-delivered programme will have higher chances of success. The most compelling learning environments are those that target the message to the audience and realize that people will learn and absorb more readily if the information is meaningful to them.

Each of these elements speaks to the necessity of positive relationships with employees, understanding their needs and having a strong corporate desire to keep human resources healthy. Disability management practitioners need to understand the impact of the organization and that they cannot operate in isolation of the corporate culture. 'In the past, the worksite health promotion field has focused on individual health. This approach has been successful for employees that choose to participate but ultimately real success can only be obtained if larger proportions of the employee population participate and improve their health behaviours. Ultimately, this will require a strategic effort to reduce health risk through a planned change approach that introduces and supports healthy behaviours' (Wilson & Wagner 1997). This by no means indicates that any one culture is the best and should be replicated; it simply proposes that a culture that understands and addresses human need will be more successful in the prevention of disability. A white-collar sales environment with highly driven 'Type A' (i.e. driven) personalities will have a very different culture than a call centre or a manufacturing shop floor. Different people and groups of people have different motivators and interests, creating different cultures and different cultural needs. The key is recognizing what motivates and what culture will support various work groups to perform optimally.

DETERMINING DISABILITY PREVENTION NEEDS

In designing health and safety and health-promotion programmes priorities should be developed based on an analysis of data. Data which can be important include short-term disability, long-term disability, workers' compensation, employee assistance plan, drug utilization and absence data. The workers' compensation data will help to identify high-risk areas that need immediate attention. The short-term and long-term disability data will give you an insight into the health of the workforce and areas where health promotion may be of value. The drug utilization data will give you an insight into future potential disability trends. The employee assistance plan data will provide aggregate information about employees' concerns and stressors. All of these data, combined with an understanding of the corporate culture, will help the DM practitioner gear programmes to the needs of the employees.

Disability prevention encompasses many important and intriguing areas including corporate culture, health and safety, and health promotion. Disability management practitioners can design and implement programmes in line with company philosophy and strategic direction to obtain optimal results. Once the incident or illness has occurred many strategies can be used to get the individual back into the workplace but none are as valuable as preventing the occurrence in the first place.

REFERENCES

Balch D 2002 Assessing health risk. Canadian Healthcare Manager, August:29–32

Biddle D, Nikki S S 1999 Protective service physical ability tests: establishing pass/fail ranking, and banding procedures. Public Personnel Management 28(2):217–225

Chaffin D B, Herrin G D, Keyserling W M 1978 Pre-employment strength testing. Journal of Occupational Medicine 20(6):403–408

Dakos M, Scott L R (2001) Post Offer Employment Testing. Paper presented at the Hanoun Medical Workshop, Toronto, Ontario, Canada, 10 October

Durand M J, Loisel P, Hong Q N et al 2002 Helping clinicians in work disability prevention: the work disability diagnosis interview. Journal of Occupational Rehabilitation 12(3):191–204

Fleishman E A 1979 Evaluating physical abilities required by jobs. The Personnel Administrator 24(6):82–91

Gilliam T B 2004 Disability on the rise in young industrial workers due to obesity epidemic – what is the cost to industry? Industrial Physical Capability Services (unpublished document)

Hogan J, Arneson S 1991 Physical and psychological assessments to reduce workers' compensation claims. In: Jones J W, Steffy B D, Bray D W (eds) Applying Psychology in Business. Lexington Books, Toronto, pp 787–801

Kirsh B 1996 Influences on the process of work integration: the consumer perspective. Canadian Journal of Community Mental Health 5:21–37

McCall M W 1998 High Flyers: Developing the next generation of leaders. Harvard Business School Press, Boston, MA

Michigan Disability Prevention Study – Research Highlights 1993 http://www.upjohninst.org/publications/wp/93-18.pdf

Nassau D W 1999 The effects of pre-work functional screening on lowering an employer's injury rate medical costs and lost workdays. Spine 24(3):269–274

Randolph D C 2000 Use of functional employment testing to facilitate safe job placement. Occupational Medicine 15(4):813–821

Scott L 2003 Measuring employee abilities. American Association of Occupational Health Nurses Journal 50(12):559–565

Wilson B, Wagner D A 1997 Developing organizational health at the worksite. American Journal of Health Studies 13(2):105–108

Chapter **6**

Programme development

LEARNING OBJECTIVES

- Understand the value of policies and procedures
- Have knowledge of how to establish policies and procedures
- Recognize the importance of appropriate roles and responsibilities
- Define the skill requirements of a disability management practitioner

INTRODUCTION

A well-developed disability management (DM) programme will have defined policy, procedures, and roles and responsibilities to govern its parameters and operation. Policies and procedures document the philosophical underpinnings of the programme, the step-by-step approach required and the detailed roles and responsibilities of the parties involved.

Policies and procedures provide the basis for programme implementation. Management has the opportunity to set policy in the workplace and should exercise this option. It removes question on how an issue will be dealt with, it establishes parameters around the programme and provides guidance to the administrators and participants. In addition it can provide consistency – even if staff changes, the premise of the policy and procedures will be continued.

POLICY TEMPLATE

Policies should have a format consistent with other workplace policies and contain at a minimum (and approved by section): title; date; revision date; and page numbers. These elements assist in confirming the policy and tracking its advancement. The organization's policy directives may also have a tone or structure that the DM policy should follow in order to align with the workplace. It is important to revisit and update these policy documents regularly (Table 6.1).

Table 6.1 Example of a policy template

	Policy and procedure
Subject	Issued by
Original date of issue	Reviewed by
Revision date	Distributed to

Policy statement

Policy statements inform the reader of the philosophical underpinnings of the programme. The statement should be brief and to the point and convey the image the company wants to portray while capturing the essence of the programme. Care must be taken to ensure that the policy statement is consistent with organizational beliefs and is aligned with the strategic direction of the corporation. To do otherwise would decrease the validity of the policy in the organization.

A well-thought-out policy statement will give the company 'philosophy and commitment' to DM, early and safe return to work (RTW), and stipulate worker and management accountability. It provides a broad guide to behaviours and the parameters of the programme. The policy will emphasize the positive impact and focus of the DM programme. A good DM programme is supportive of production values in recognizing that employees are valuable to the organization, that worker participation is valued and that the workplace is responsive to the workers' needs.

Procedures

Procedures provide the venue for a presentation of the programme in a step-by-step manner. Disability management requires specific actions to be successful:

- immediate reporting
- early communication
- contact with the healthcare providers
- return-to-work philosophy and prompt offer of RTW solutions
- conflict resolution options
- evaluation and continuous improvement.

Each of these elements requires an understanding of the organization and its structure to be effective and efficient.

Immediate reporting

In work-related conditions there is a legislative requirement to report immediately. In non-occupational situations the requirements may vary by worksite but generally an elapsed-day trigger will be set (for example, absences of over three days will require the employee to submit sufficient medical evidence). This trigger helps distinguish between 'absence' and 'disability' and should be specified in the procedure. The procedure should also specify when, how and who the employee should report to following a disability.

Early communication

It is essential in a DM programme to have early communication with the absent employee. The contact must convey genuine concern and be supportive in nature (Bernacki & Tsai 2003, Krause et al 1998, Larsson & Gard 2003). This step should be adequately conveyed in the procedures.

Contact with the healthcare providers

Healthcare providers are not the gatekeepers in DM. However, they can provide important information about the current health status and recovery projection for the worker. The objective of the contact is to obtain abilities information and determine if the employee has any needs or requirements to expedite RTW. The DM practitioner will perform the job match in conjunction with the workplace and the employee based on this information.

Return-to-work philosophy and prompt offer of return-to-work solutions

Return-to-work availability is pivotal to the DM process and an essential step in the procedures. Return to work is a process specific to the individual's needs and should include a joint meeting to formulate a RTW plan (Adams & Williams 2003, Baril et al 2003, Blackwell et al 2003, Friesen et al 2001). Elements that need to be considered in the planning of RTW are:

- Is RTW mandatory when suitable modified work is available?
- Does the work have to be in the employee's previous work area or can it be anywhere the work is available?
- What is the expected and maximum duration of modified work and what happens when that maximum is reached?
- How is the employee compensated while on modified work?
- When and how is permanent impairment accommodation initiated?

Return to work has been a primary focus of DM programmes and may require several steps in the procedure.

Conflict resolution options

Regardless of the programme there will be occasions when conflict arises. It is important to have a process in place to delineate the steps and key responsibilities for conflict resolution in advance. In unionized organizations, with collective agreements and grievance procedures in place, it is possible to use existing avenues to deal with disputes or develop an agreed-upon resolution pattern for DM and RTW issues.

Evaluation and continuous improvement

The measuring of outcomes and development of continuous improvement methods is essential to any DM programme. This aspect will assist in identifying areas to fine tune the programme and meet the needs of workplace parties. This aspect should be ingrained in the procedures.

Procedures will commence with the event of injury or illness, discuss case management, RTW, dispute resolution/appeals, evaluation measures and continuous improvement methods. These establish a consistent method of accomplishing the DM process and help to ensure that all staff are using a standard approach (Amann 2001).

Roles and responsibilities

The roles and responsibilities of those who administrate or interact with the programme need to be defined. While the procedures provide a step-by-step summary of activities, the roles and responsibilities outline what roles key individuals play in order to make the programme operate successfully. At a minimum the participants include the employee, DM practitioner and supervisors. Others may include human resources, unions, treating healthcare practitioners, preferred provider organizations, third-party administrators, insurer, Workers' Compensation Board or Insurer, and management. Many individuals may be involved in the day-to-day administration of DM programmes at the worksite or in the development of the RTW plan with the employee. Roles may also vary and evolve depending on the size of the workplace, the employee's unique circumstances and the infrastructure that exists.

The breakdown of the roles and responsibilities most often defined in DM are:

- injured or ill employee
- disability management practitioner
- healthcare providers or preferred providers
- management – supervisor, manager, etc.
- benefit adjudication providers – insurance company, third-party administrator, workers' compensation
- employee representatives or union (if applicable).

Injured or ill employee

The employee is the primary individual in the process. He or she will always have the obligation to report the injury or illness, complete the required paperwork, maintain contact with the employer, provide documentation, participate in treatment to recover and participate in the RTW programme.

Disability management practitioner

The DM practitioner could be human resources, an occupational health nurse, a RTW coordinator, or other designate in the workplace or external to the workplace. The key responsibilities of this individual can vary depending on the workplace structure. However, they could include:

- assisting in disability prevention and health promotion activities
- providing the employee with information about DM process
- submitting a claim in cases of illness or injury
- maintaining close contact with the employee while off work
- solving problems in difficult case situations
- communicating with external agencies such as workers' compensation, insurer or third-party administrator
- identifying the potential for RTW
- communicating with workplace supervisors, co-workers, union members, healthcare providers and community groups
- arranging for assessments, e.g. medical, ergonomic, rehabilitation
- selecting and monitoring preferred provider organizations
- assisting with the transition back to work: regular; modified; or rehabilitative
- educating the workforce on the importance of DM programmes
- maintaining the confidentiality of employee records
- establishing goals and objectives for the programme
- collecting and evaluating information to monitor the success of the programme
- communicating the programme outcomes
- providing knowledge transfer on the programme parameters.

Healthcare providers and preferred providers

Healthcare providers have a role in ensuring that the employee receives the right treatment necessary to recover. They also have an obligation to provide information on the capabilities of the worker when RTW is being planned.

Management – supervisor, manager, etc.

Management has a responsibility to provide a safe working environment. Supervisors play a central role in DM, and their support of RTW is essential to make the programme a success. Also, they should stay in touch with the employee to maintain the connection with the workplace. Management should work closely with the DM practitioner and the employee to design RTW that is suitable to the employee's capabilities. The supervisor plays an important role in the control of other workplace responses such as co-worker support of the returning employee. It is important to bear in mind the health and safety of co-workers when facilitating RTW that requires adjustment of the worker's task (Larsson & Gard 2003) and not unnecessarily burden other workers, thereby increasing their risk of injury. Co-worker response is an important ingredient in successful RTW (Wassel 2002) and supervisors can ensure that co-workers understand the necessity of modified work, its availability to all members of the workforce, and support the individual positively in their transition back to full duties.

Senior management should show visible support for the programme and its objectives. They should endorse accountability at every level to ensure that the programme is being delivered in accordance with procedures.

Benefit adjudication providers – insurance company, third-party administrator, workers' compensation

These external parties play an essential role in promoting and supporting early and safe RTW. Generally, there are contracts or legislation that guide their behaviours. Contracts should be reviewed to ensure that early and safe RTW is supported. In cases when return to the former employer is not possible these providers play a very important role in facilitating appropriate rehabilitation sooner rather than later.

Employee representatives or union (if applicable)

In workplaces with unions or employee representatives it is important that this group convey visible support for the programme. Disability management is a positive programme for employees, thus the union's membership, if handled properly, has many benefits. A union's role will include promoting the DM philosophy, early and safe RTW, and working with the company to ensure that safe RTW is possible.

POLICY AND PROCEDURE MANUAL

Once the manual has been developed it is important to have it reviewed by the key participants in the DM process. This will ensure that senior management (and union leaders if applicable) are aware of – and have an opportunity to provide – input into the final product. The manual may have been developed by the DM practitioner or by a DM committee assembled by the workplace for this task. Either way a final review is essential to ensure success.

However, the project is not over once the manual is produced. It is not a publication to sit on the shelf; it is meant to guide workplace behaviours in DM and should be reviewed regularly. Additionally, periodic reviews to maintain currency with legislation and other adjunct workplace policies will be necessary.

Communication of the final product is vital to its success. Management sessions, supervisor sessions and employee sessions are all key in the roll-out phase. The DM procedures should also be built into the orientation programme.

Implementing the programme

If the programme already exists it is a matter of ensuring that the appropriate documentation is in place and that there is continual communication of the programme. If it is a new disability programme a development and communication strategy should be developed.

One of the first important elements is to ensure buy-in from executive senior management. The executive team support will add credibility to the programme but most importantly it will assist if 'roadblocks' occur. This support will be invaluable. Executive support can mean the difference between a programme being implemented or shelved. A business case may need to be formulated using baseline data to support the necessity and value of the programme or ongoing data. It will help emphasize the value of the programme, the advantages and the potential bottom-line impact. Success measures and any resources required should be explored and included in the change management strategy or communication plan.

Once executive buy-in is established the management team should be made familiar with the programme and the benefits. Management should be prepared to convey their support for the programme to the supervisors and workers.

Supervisors

Supervisors will require an overview of the programme – the whys, hows and whens. Most importantly they will need to be aware of their roles in the process. It is important to develop simple tools for supervisors to use in the event of disability. Supervisor training sessions will be an integral part of the launch of the programme. Its details should be built into the orientation programme and the annual training plan.

Union

The union needs to be aware of the programme prior to implementation so any issues or concerns can be dealt with prior to implementation. The programme is a positive benefit for the membership and, if positioned properly within the functioning structure, the organization's labour/management style will be perceived positively. Some organizations may choose to establish a joint committee to establish the programme if this is within their usual labour or management structure and style. Other organizations may choose to inform the union and ask for input prior to and during the implementation. Other organizations may view DM as a management initiative and proceed directly to implementation of the programme.

Employee

Employee communication is important so that, if an illness or injury occurs, they know what to do. Disability management is a positive benefit: it conveys to employees that the company will not abandon them during periods of illness or injury. It lets employees know that they are valued. The communication plan can be as simple as a brochure included with pay stubs, through to posters on bulletin boards, to full-blown employee communication. Again, this will depend on whether the programme is new or existing and the usual communication style of the company. The most important point to convey is who employees must contact if they ever need programme details.

In workplaces where the DM practitioner participates with other health and safety, environment and human resources management groups' specific discussions with these close affiliations should occur to align process and communication. Many of these individuals may have already been involved in the development process.

Ultimately, the communication plan will be guided by company culture and should emphasize the 'What's in it for me' to each group.

Benchmarking and best practices

In the field of DM there are known international evidence-based best practices. These should be incorporated into procedures and practices.

It is important that policies and procedures are living documents, and as continuous improvement areas are identified they are incorporated into the procedures. Programmes should evolve as improvements are made in the company and as research on proven strategies continue to become more sophisticated.

DISABILITY MANAGEMENT – INTERNAL OR EXTERNAL MODEL

Disability management may be based on an internal or external model or a combination of both. Each organization has to make its own decisions as to whether they wish to hire and support internal expertise or purchase external expertise. There are advantages to both models.

A company with internal DM has the practitioner immediately on site to deal with each issue as it arises; there is direct management control over the DM practitioner's activities and priority response to emergency situations.

The external model has the advantage of having a group of experts that hold DM as their core competency. External DM practitioners are less likely to be drawn into internal politics or agendas and will make decisions based on evidence best practices and the merits of the case. External DM firms have multiple resources to ensure that they stay up-to-date on recent research on DM. The internal versus external decision can be impacted by the size of the company, the location of the company, the definition of core competencies and past experience.

It is not uncommon to see a combination approach that uses the best of both elements. Some internal resources may be used while some external components may also be used for areas that require specific expertise.

When selecting an external vendor there are a number of key considerations:

- vision and cultural fit
- disability management technical expertise
- staff qualifications
- quality assurance methods
- outcome measures
- continuous improvement approach
- fees.

Vision and cultural fit

The external firm must understand the needs of the organization. Each firm and its key contacts have a philosophy and it is important that this matches with the company. An understanding of this element is essential to a productive relationship.

Disability management technical expertise

It is important to ensure that the firm being hired to perform the external case management has the technical expertise to accomplish the objectives of the DM programme. This would include knowledge of DM principles and processes that have been proven as effective in their implementation as based on evidence-based research.

Staff qualifications

Technical expertise is one of the key reasons for an external model. It is important that the staff working on the account have the right qualifications and commitment. It is important to exercise caution when hiring an external firm and to ensure that one understands their own internal hiring practices. The employees should be qualified, experienced, knowledgeable and have an employment relationship with the DM firm. If the external provider has contractors or individuals with little experience, their potential to administer effectively will be diminished and the company will not achieve the desired outcomes.

Quality assurance methods

The importance of the quality assurance methods of the external provider cannot be underestimated. There needs to be a structured approach towards ensuring quality interventions and the maintenance of confidentiality.

Outcome measures

Tracking and evaluation are clearly important measures in either internal or external models. Time, effort and money go into the implementation of DM programmes, and evidence-based research includes the positive quantitative and qualitative benefits of DM interventions. Interventions and outcomes need to be measured and communicated to the company in an adequate manner.

Continuous improvement approach

The outcomes of the programme evaluation will assist with the development of continuous improvement mechanisms. Continuous improvement is a key ingredient for success in any organization.

Fees

Competitive fees are always important in external relationships. However, companies need to ensure that fees are adequate to cover the expected level of service, and that there is no underbidding to acquire the account but then an inability to deliver.

DISABILITY MANAGEMENT PRACTITIONER QUALIFICATIONS

The DM practitioner, whether internal or external to the organization, must have appropriate knowledge, skills and capabilities to perform the role. Typically, the ideal candidate will possess:

- a university degree with additional certification in DM or occupational health and safety
- 5–10 years of experience in occupational health or DM with progression of knowledge, skills and responsibilities
- knowledge of pertinent legislation and evidence-based best practices
- strong communication skills
- computer ability
- business acumen.

Education

It is essential to hire DM practitioners who at least have a basic knowledge of the theory behind DM techniques. Many educational programmes exist to help DM practitioners acquire education in this area.

Experience

As in many professions, practical experience is essential to understand the finer points of the profession. Every situation will be unique and require different approaches to ultimately resolve the disability, especially when interacting with employees. When hiring, experience is an important element and progression of skills and job responsibilities is a good sign that the experience has resulted in positive outcomes.

Knowledge

Disability management practitioners need to be familiar with legislation and its influence on the DM process. There is an expectation that knowledge will be sought in areas of legislation, professional advances and evidence-based research. The DM practitioner should have a level of recognition for the value for continuous learning.

Communication skills

Communication skills are essential in DM. Some of the important components of communication are an ability to articulate thoughts concisely and factually, an understanding of confidentiality principles, data collection and analysis skills, report writing capability, presentation skills, and proficient listening and persuasion skills.

Computer ability

Many tasks are performed on the computer including data gathering, data generation and case tracking. Electronic communication has become one of the essential components of every job; ability must exist in this area to be a DM practitioner.

Business skills

Disability management has a direct influence on corporation and business skills including planning, organizing, decision-making, leadership, financial ability, conflict resolution and change management. An important element in any DM programme is knowing how to perform change management effectively.

CONCLUSION

Disability management policy, procedures, and roles and responsibilities are important elements in high-functioning DM programmes. The design of policy and procedures convey senior management support and direction for the implementation of the programme. Roles and responsibilities define everyone's part in the effective operation of the programme, ensuring that no steps are missed and the programme has a basis for efficient execution.

REFERENCES

Adams J H, Williams A 2003 What affects return to work for graduates of a pain-management program with chronic upper limb pain. Journal of Occupational Rehabilitation 13(2):91–106

Amann M 2001 The policy and procedure manual – keeping it current. American Association of Occupational Health Nurses 49(2):69–71

Baril R, Berthelette D, Massicotte P 2003 Early return to work of injured workers: multidimensional patterns of individual and organizational factors. Safety Science 41: 277–300

Bernacki E J, Tsai S P 2003 Ten years experience using an integrated Workers' Compensation management system to control workers' compensation costs. Journal of Occupational and Environmental Medicine 45(5):508–516

Blackwell T L, Leierer S J, Haupt S et al 2003 Predictors of vocational rehabilitation return to work outcomes in Workers' Compensation. Rehabilitation Counseling Bulletin 46(2):108–114

Friesen M N, Yassi A, Cooper J 2001 Return to work: the importance of human interactions and organizational structure. Work 17:11–22

Krause N, Dasinger L K, Neuhauser F 1998 Modified work and return to work: a review of the literature. Journal of Occupational Rehabilitation 82:113–139

Larsson A, Gard G 2003 How can rehabilitation planning process at the workplace be improved? A qualitative study from employers' perspective. Journal of Occupational Rehabilitation 13(3):169–181

Wassel M L 2002 Improving return to work outcomes. Formalizing the process. American Association of Occupational Health Nurses Journal 50(6):275–285

Chapter **7**

Early intervention

INTRODUCTION

The concept of early intervention can be traced back in the general rehabilitation literature to the 1950s. During this time the United Nations attempted to refocus treatment from clinical settings to the workplace. However, all efforts were focused on individuals with chronic or permanent functional limitations. No thought was given to what we now refer to as temporary injuries or disabilities. As any practitioner today knows, it is this latter type of condition that is the cost driver in today's rehabilitation systems.

Early intervention has an important role to play in this population in that social and psychological concerns often outweigh physical concerns and these in turn form major barriers to successful return to work (RTW). In order to be effective in their work, disability management (DM) practitioners need to understand the concepts that underlie effective early intervention and what to do in order to ensure that early intervention results in a successful return to work.

In an earlier publication one of the authors (Harder 2003) referred to the period post-injury as 'traumatically induced unemployment'. It is important to understand that individuals who are away from work due to an injury or illness undergo the same reactions and consequences as people who are unemployed due, for example, to a plant closure. We know from the results of many studies that work is part of establishing and maintaining a healthy identity and that prolonged unemployment can lead to severe psychological distress. This distress results from factors such as loss of income, loss of a work identity, loss of social support and loss of a daily structure. When someone is off work due to an injury or illness most, if not all, of these factors begin to apply. The longer the person is off work the more severe the impact of these issues becomes.

For example, Mr C was a 52-year-old office worker who had been employed with the same employer for over 20 years. Mr C was single (never married) and made extensive use of the employer's social activities. He was a member of the curling club, social club, etc. He also ate two meals a day in the employer's cafeteria and ate dinner out. He had very limited social contact outside work and stated that his only purpose in life was to go to work.

Mr C sustained an injury that caused him to be away from work. Initially, no one from the employer contacted him and he was left at home alone. Quite apart from his injury, his physical health deteriorated as he had never learned to cook for himself. Many weeks passed and by the time he was contacted he was bitter and well on the way to depression. When the RTW process began he was angry, resistant and proved to be a difficult case. It is important to note that this difficulty had nothing to do with the physical after-effects of his injury. He felt betrayed by his employer and his friends. He was questioning why he should return to work in an environment that did not value him. All of this could have been avoided if he had been contacted at an appropriate time, if the worksite had maintained contact, and possibly provided some minor assistance to him throughout his recovery, all of which is part of early intervention in DM.

What happens to someone like Mr C when they are away from work? One common development is that they slip into depression. It is usual for people to feel 'blue' when recovering from an injury. However, this feeling can rapidly turn into a sense of hopelessness and then depression. According to the DSM IV (American Psychiatric Association 1994), depression is characterized by factors such as:

- depressed mood most of the day
- markedly diminished interest or pleasure in all, or almost all, activities
- significant weight gain or loss
- insomnia or hypersomnia (excessive sleep)
- psychomotor agitation or retardation
- fatigue or loss of energy
- diminished ability to think or concentrate
- indecisiveness
- at the extreme, recurrent thoughts of death and/or suicide.

A person has to meet at least five of these criteria to be diagnosed with depression. How can such a person return to work? The answer is with great difficulty. Empirical evidence suggests that people who are depressed and who are inactive and pessimistic in their outlook will stay unemployed much longer than those who are not (Frese & Mohr 1987). At this stage there is very little that a DM practitioner can do as this person will require treatment for their depression before the RTW process can be started. It is therefore of great importance that the DM practitioner intervene early, before depression can begin.

LEARNED HELPLESSNESS

Where does depression come from? One concept that can help us understand the development of depression is the construct of learned helplessness as first promulgated by Seligman (1975). Learned helplessness is caused by repeated experiences of aversive, non-controllable situations. A person caught up in learned helplessness exhibits passive, resigned, inflexible behaviour, linked to feelings of depression brought on as a result of repeating these situations. The only escape is to exercise control over these situations. For example, Ms E is a delivery driver who is injured in a motor vehicle accident while working; the other driver was not working. Ms E was not at fault. However, she had a previous Workers' Compensation Board (WCB) claim for the same part of the body. The WCB and the other driver's insurance company are arguing over who should pay for her rehabilitation and lost wages. In the meantime she is left to wait at home. She makes repeated attempts to contact adjusters from both organizations explaining her physical and financial needs. She is always told not to worry and that they will work it out soon. She is very dissatisfied, desperate for money and tries many times to move things forward. However, after being repeatedly rebuffed she gives up, stays at home and starts watching daytime TV as a way to escape the turmoil that the loss of a pay cheque is causing her family. She lies on the couch feeling totally helpless. Hopelessness and depression are waiting in the wings.

LOCUS OF CONTROL

Another concept useful in understanding the aetiology of depression is the notion of locus of control. Locus of control simply asks the question: who is in control of my life anyway? Me or them? In the early descriptions of this concept a two-dimensional model was described. In this model it was generally believed that the external locus of control was bad and internal was good. It was posited that people with an external locus of control tend to blame others for their experiences, exhibit passive behaviour and do not take responsibility for their own actions. Persons with an internal locus of control make sense of their experiences from the perspective of their own actions and thoughts. They tend to take action and try to alter their experiences. This two-dimensional understanding seems too simplistic and we suggest that there are at least two more dimensions as illustrated below, and that people move between the dimensions. This is summarized in Table 7.1.

Given the difficulty inherent in working with someone in the two negative quadrants it is imperative that we intervene early enough to avoid the slide from positive to negative. Some individuals will be in one of the negative quadrants prior to injury. In such cases, referral to an appropriate professional such as a psychologist may be in order.

A frequent example of the progression from positive to negative is when someone is injured as a result of a safety violation. The injured worker most likely feels that there was nothing they could do. If the employer does not

Table 7.1 Locus of control model

Internal positive	Internal negative
• Accepts appropriate responsibility • Takes action	• Blames themselves by taking too much responsibility • Is stuck; may lash out
External positive	**External negative**
• Accepts the existence of a higher being • Consults and takes direction from valued others • Moves forward once consultation is completed	• Blames others • Takes no responsibility for their own actions • Waits for others to fix things for them

act quickly to remedy the safety issue then the worker will feel helpless and begin to blame others for his or her situation. If this is allowed to continue the individual will soon be in a negative external locus of control position.

PERSONAL CONSTRUCTS

A third concept that allows us to understand how a person slips into depression is that of the personal construct. A personal construct is a transparent pattern that individuals use to organize the realities of their world. Individuals create constructs by deciding what theme is common in two or more events. This common theme is determined through a process of comparing and contrasting events until a similarity is found between at least two of these events. Personal constructs are developed over time, as a result of personal experience, and are formed into systems. Constructs provide a window or lens through which people perceive and understand events and also supply a mechanism for anticipating events and experiences. For example, suppose that a woman notices that her supervisor is more irritable at the end of the working week than at the beginning of the week. She has a construct that enables her to recognize irritability. She may also use related constructs, such as more rest on the weekend and time to participate in relaxing activities, as she attempts to interpret her experience with her supervisor and anticipate future interaction. Forster (1992) selected the personal construct as the 'primary conceptual unit for investigating the elicitation and articulation of a person's goals' (p 176).

Kelly (1955), the creator of personal construct theory, believed that vocational development 'is one of the principal means by which one's life role is given clarity and meaning' (p 751). Construct systems developed by individuals in the course of their work experiences are called vocational construct systems. Such systems might contain constructs like outdoor work, desk jobs, high wages or low salary. Individuals would use these constructs to organize and systematize their work experiences and to anticipate future employment experiences. Gimenes (1990) assigned the label of vocational development construct to the interaction of:

1. The factors that motivate people to form vocational construct systems.
2. The elements that prevent people from forming vocational construct systems.
3. The factors that trigger specific employment decisions.

Since vocational development is based on work experience and all previous vocational decisions, Gimenes concluded that the construct clearly indicated that selecting an occupational goal is a complex process that takes time.

Evidence of some relationship between level of integration in personal construct systems and decision-making has implications for the design of programmes that include the identification of skills based on previous experience and the selection of new goals. Successful RTW post-injury may require higher levels of integration of personal construct systems. All people – but particularly those faced with the reality of having to make substantial efforts in order to return to work – must reorganize their personal construct systems to incorporate both the experience of injury and recovery and the personal constructs that will guide their decision-making throughout their treatment and the RTW process.

Everyone who is employed has a personal construct of themselves as a worker. When they are injured this begins to change to that of an injured worker, and then if all goes well, to a recovering worker and eventually a recovered 'back-at-the-job' worker. All too frequently, as a result of lack of intervention or long delay in intervention, the construct changes from worker to benefits recipient, to angry benefits recipient, to 'cut-off-benefits' angry individual, to advocate for rights, to no worker construct whatsoever. An early intervention stops this progression and keeps the focus on work and enables the worker to maintain their worker personal construct.

The following is a real case that demonstrates the consequences of the lack of early and appropriate intervention. Ms M was a mother of three young children all in various sports and activities as well as school. They lived on a hobby farm and raised horses. Every morning Ms M and her husband were up before dawn cleaning out stalls, grooming and feeding the horses. Then it was the children's turn, and off to school and work. She had a very demanding job, dealing with customer complaints at a large retail outlet, but she loved it, by all accounts was good at it and had an excellent employment record. She had no record of previous serious illness or injuries. After work the children were taken by one parent or another to various activities, before homework, lights out and sleep. Clearly Ms M had many constructs in operation. There is the construct of mother, driver, worker, organizer, horse person, etc. Perhaps the most important to her, by her own admission, was the vocational construct of a very well-functioning, well-organized, capable woman.

One day, while transporting the children, their van was hit broadside in an intersection. Ms M was not at fault. The children were alright but Ms M received a very nasty bump and bruise to the left side of her head where she had hit the front pillar. Initially all was well. Then she began having vision and balance problems. At work she was curt and increasingly intolerant of others. At home she was fatigued, irritable and neglected her responsibilities. She was diagnosed as having a mild traumatic brain injury. By the time she was referred to a DM practitioner a little over a year had elapsed. It was far too late for early intervention. By that time she was no longer working and barely functional. Her husband had taken over most of the responsibilities and was not happy about it. She was clinically depressed and referred to a psychologist who worked with her for a while and she began to recover. She was ready to attempt a return to work when the insurance companies involved began preparing for court and she was sent for neuropsychological evaluation. Both sides of the case wanted different assessments and, inevitably, the assessments did not agree. Ms M did not take all of the assessments very well and concluded that the insurance companies simply did not believe her. Her further conclusion based on that assumption was that she had to forget about going back to work and had to concentrate on fighting for her rights and the rights of others like her.

Let's examine the case of Ms M. Why was there no early intervention? Early intervention did not occur largely because the claims manager involved assumed she would get better on her own. He did not want to use up resources if she was going to recover anyway. However, there were plenty of warnings that this was not going to be a basic and easy case. All these markers were ignored until it was too late. Then the insurance company went into loss-prevention mode, trying to limit their financial exposure and attacking the credibility of Ms M. This type of 'penny wise, pound foolish' approach is not uncommon in the insurance industry and is one reason why insurance costs are on the increase as insurance companies try to reduce costs in the courts rather than early in the claim, where a few 'pennies' spent would potentially save many 'pounds' later.

As there was no early intervention Ms M was left to her own devices; she quickly learned that she was essentially on her own. She had an extremely frustrating relationship with her claims adjuster and quickly drifted into learned helplessness. It also became apparent that she had moved into the external negative quadrant but had some internal positive left in her in that she believed that she could get better and back to the life she loved. Finally, her personal and vocational constructs were destroyed and replaced first with a 'poor me' victim construct but then with an advocacy construct. The whole experience of the legal system had a skewed effect on her. While she strengthened her internal positive quadrant, developed a new personal construct and moved out of the learned helplessness position, all of this change was not directed at work or personal activities. It was directed at getting even with the system and getting what was due to her. Arguably this is an improvement but hardly one that we are striving to attain.

Ms M may be an extreme case but lesser versions of her experience occur on a regular basis. Early intervention must become and remain a priority of all systems that work with injured or ill people. Delays have very serious and often life-altering consequences. Proper early assistance would go a long way towards ensuring that people such as Ms M return successfully to their lives post-injury or -illness.

EARLY INTERVENTION

Our understanding of early intervention has changed markedly over the years. From 'early rehabilitation', which suggested that physical rehabilitation could occur before physical recovery had been achieved, to 'early intervention', which suggested that rehabilitation services could happen much sooner in the process and perhaps even at the worksite, to the DM view of early intervention, which is that all possible assistance required, whether physical, emotional, financial, etc., be provided as soon as possible in order to help the person return to the worksite as soon as feasible.

In the case of psychological and non-physiological claims, early intervention should occur prior to the person leaving the worksite and can include tactics such as ergonomic or environmental assessments whose intent is to intervene early enough to be able to implement corrective or helping measures that will keep the person in the workforce. Keeping people at the worksite by preventing illness or injury is the ultimate form of early intervention.

The steps of early intervention case management are:

1. Make contact just to let them know about your support:
   a. If appropriate, get the claims process under way, forms, etc.
   b. Ensure that they will not 'drop off of the radar'
2. Monitor physical recovery and treatment processes:
   a. Ensure that physical treatment is going along as it should. This does not mean that you are taking the place of the physician. You are simply ensuring that there are no systemic delays preventing them from getting timely and appropriate treatment
3. Set the stage to stay in frequent contact with the worker:
   a. Make sure that they understand that you are there to help them return to work.

Initial contact

It is imperative that contact be made as early as possible, given the parameters of human decency post-injury or the onset of disease. Once a condition has been determined not to be life-threatening, the thoughts of the individual and the family usually turn to matters of financial security. One of the first questions asked is: how will we survive without an income? The DM practitioner should be ready to discuss what benefits the person may be entitled to and how these will be accessed. Any necessary forms should be filled out and sent to the correct source at the insurance company, third-party administrator or workers' compensation authority. Many cases begin to go wrong at this very early stage as forms are mislaid, misdirected or incorrectly filled out. As critical as this is, the main goal of this contact is to ensure that the injured or ill individual and their family understand that the organization cares for them, sees them as a valued employee and will stand by them during their recovery and RTW process. By taking this step early in the process we ensure that the person feels valued, knows they will get the best care possible, is expected to return to work and will be assisted in this process. This will prevent the person from becoming bitter as a result of being neglected or as we often hear 'being cast on the waste heap'. Such bitterness often results in reluctance or outright refusal to cooperate in the RTW process. A cared-for person, who knows from the outset that return to work is expected once they have recovered, is much more likely to return to work successfully and more quickly.

Monitoring

Many things can go wrong in the course of a person's recovery period. Delays inherent in the health system can hold up treatment, causing complications. Diagnostic assessments such as MRI can be delayed for long periods, causing great confusion and anxiety. Physicians and insurance adjusters can disagree on what type of assessment or treatment should be offered. The family system can realign around a disability causing a change in the motivation to get better. These are just a few examples of what can go wrong and why it is extremely important for the DM practitioner to stay in regular and frequent contact with the injured or ill worker. The earlier a problem is identified the earlier a solution can be applied. It is the DM practitioner's job to ensure that all aspects of the recovery go as smoothly as possible.

For example, Mr D is at home awaiting a CT scan appointment. He has been told that, due to a lengthy waiting list, it will be at least three months before he can have the scan. When, during a weekly call, the DM practitioner discovers this an immediate call is made to the hospital. As the practitioner suspected, as a result of previous experience, an almost immediate CT scan is available if the person is willing to come in at odd hours or at short notice of a cancellation. The practitioner calls the worker and explains the situation. The CT scan is performed the following week. It seems ludicrous that no one at the healthcare facility would have explained this to the worker. In our experience, however, this is quite common, especially for people who are having their wages covered through an insurance plan. It appears that healthcare providers simply believe that these people can wait, not understanding how they are damaging both the person and the insurance provider through such action. Because of their extensive knowledge of the system and by taking action based on this knowledge, the practitioner can often ensure that the person gains timely access to services that might be otherwise delayed.

It is very important that the practitioner realizes and accepts that he or she is not stepping into the role of a physician or other healthcare provider. It is not the practitioner's job to second guess a medical opinion or the direction of the treatment – it is the practitioner's job to ensure that no systemic delays interfere with the worker's recovery.

Regular contact

No matter how long the recovery period is, it is vital that the DM practitioner stays in regular contact, not only for the reasons outlined above but also to ensure that social contact is maintained with the worksite and to maintain the expectation that the worker will return to work as soon as possible. It is critical to the worker's emotional wellbeing, and eventual successful return to work, that contact with the worksite be maintained. In fact, the longer the worker is away the more critical it becomes. Many people feel uncomfortable returning to work after a holiday, largely because there is uncertainty in what they will encounter on that first day back. Now imagine the anxiety felt by someone who has been away from work for months and has had no contact with the worksite. The DM practitioner can ease some of this anxiety by providing information on what is happening at work, reassuring the person that their job is still available to them, perhaps even encouraging the person to have coffee with their workmates once they are fit to do so. This regular contact will provide reassurance, allowing the person to focus on their recovery and encouraging them to look forward to the time when they will return to work.

CONCLUSION

Appropriate, timely emphasis on early intervention is critical in ensuring that people with acquired disabilities are able to return to work and resume their normal activities of daily living. Too long a delay, measured in only days not weeks, can lead to some very dire if unintentional consequences. As has been shown in this chapter, there are a number of sound psychological concepts that explain what happens to a person who is left alone for too long. Disability management programmes and DM professionals must continue to advocate for all systems – medical, insurance, human resources, labour – to embrace the principles of early intervention. Of course, there is such a thing as too early intervention. It is imperative that intervention occurs at the correct time but as early as appropriate. It is not alright to set an intervention timeframe that allows for all manner of time delays to be considered such as 'we'll intervene at three months because by then it should be OK'. Such programme rules are ill-advised. Early intervention requires an individualized approach, i.e. individualized to the person, to their medical and rehabilitation needs, to their employment situation, to their workplace's needs and to the needs of the insurer. Every person and every case is unique, and every case and every person benefits from early intervention.

REFERENCES

American Psychiatric Association 1994 Diagnostic and Statistical Manual of Mental Disorders, 4th edn (DSM-IV). American Psychiatric Association, Washington, DC

Forster J R 1992 Eliciting personal constructs and articulating goals. Journal of Career Development 18:175–185

Frese M, Mohr G 1987 Prolonged unemployment and depression in older workers: a longitudinal study of intervening variables. Social Science Medicine 25:173–178

Gimenes M G 1990 Theoretical perspectives. In: Schiro-Geist C (ed) Vocational Counseling for Special Populations. Charles C Thomas, Springfield, IL, pp 19–43

Harder H G 2003 Early intervention in disability management: factors that influence successful return to work. International Journal of Disability, Community and Rehabilitation 2(2):1–8

Kelly G A 1955 The Psychology of Personal Constructs, Vol 1, 2. W W Norton, New York, p 751

Seligman M E P 1975 Helplessness: On depression, development and death. Freeman, San Francisco

Chapter 8

Claim initiation

LEARNING OBJECTIVES

- Understand the claim initiation and submission processes for occupational and non-occupational claims
- Know when and how to initiate disability claims
- Define the differences between occupational and non-occupational claims
- Recognize the importance of appropriate claim-initiation methods
- Understand potential offsets

INTRODUCTION

Claim initiation is the first step in the claims process when an employee experiences occupational or non-occupational illness or injury. Work-related injuries are generally submitted to a Workers' Compensation Insurer or Workers' Compensation Board if the employer is covered by workers' compensation. On the non-occupational side of disability there are a variety of mechanisms for claiming non-occupational benefits for injury or illness. They range from government-administered to employer-sponsored benefits.

ENTITLEMENT TO BENEFITS

It should be noted that the breadth of benefits varies by country and also by region within the country. The disability management (DM) practitioner needs to be familiar with the legislation governing the country and province or state where they work.

Most developed nations have some sort of income replacement plan for work-related situations. The entitlement to these benefits is based on whether or not the individual's disability arose out of work-related activities. Companies are 100% responsible for the cost of workers' compensation coverage and submit a premium to the appropriate insurer or Workers' Compensation Board to have this coverage. Workers' compensation was established in the early 1900s to provide wage replacement and reimbursement for medical costs for those injured at work. The premise is that workers' compensation coverage is a no-fault philosophy. This eliminates the threat of the employee suing the employer for damages under tort law in exchange for guaranteed coverage for work-related injury or illness. While not all companies have to participate in workers' compensation programmes, generally those in positions requiring physical labour conditions have mandatory coverage. If a work-related incident occurs, the employer, employee and treating physician must file a claim with the Workers' Compensation Board or Insurer.

A study by Shannon and Lowe (2002) indicated that in the USA and Canada about 30% of lost-time claimants did not submit a claim. Surveys suggested that it was easier and quicker to file with the workplace sickness and disability plan. This is an interesting finding as the majority of sick-leave plans exclude work-related disabilities, stipulating that the employee must file with workers' compensation.

If there is no workers' compensation coverage or if the condition is not work-related then the employee may apply for other government-administered or employer-sponsored disability programmes, as available. The availability of non-work-related disability programmes will vary by employer and country of residence. Countries such as Canada have an employment insurance disability programme that will provide some loss of earnings benefit during illness for a period of 15 weeks with a two-week waiting period. Employers pay for this programme jointly with employees through payroll deductions and submissions.

In serious and prolonged disability cases, Canada Pension Plan (CPP) disability benefit or USA social security benefit may be an option following the initial 17 weeks of disability. Again, employers and employees share the cost of funding this programme through payroll deductions and submissions. Eligibility may depend on many factors such as employment status (part-time or full-time), duration of employment, seniority, severity of the condition, duration of contributions to the plan, etc. This benefit has to be applied for by completing the required government paperwork and submitting it to the appropriate government office. The government agency then makes a decision on whether the disability qualifies for coverage under the parameters of the legislation. If the decision on disability payments is negative the employee has the opportunity to appeal against this decision and continue to seek benefits under this programme.

If the disability is as a result of a motor vehicle accident, coverage may be pursued through the automobile insurance carrier if there is a loss of earnings. In circumstances where there is an employer disability plan, in the majority of cases the employer's plan will be the first payer.

If none of the above are suitable options there may be a variety of other social programmes that could assist the employee financially, such as government welfare programmes.

The above procedures are summarized in Figure 8.1.

Non-occupational plans

Employer-sponsored plans may have a waiting period or seniority requirement. The employee may have to work for the employer for at least three

Figure 8.1 Claim initiation flowchart.

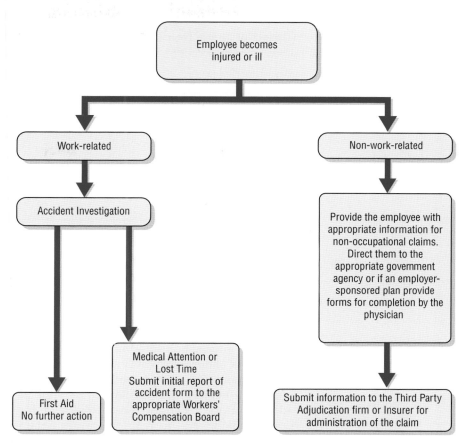

or six months prior to qualifying for employer-sponsored benefits programmes. Waiting periods are commonly three to five days prior to disability benefits commencing.

Sick leave plans

If the employer has a sick leave or salary continuance plan, employees can apply for benefits through this by submitting appropriate paperwork including information from their physicians with sufficient medical evidence to support their disabilities. Benefits may last for casual absence of short duration, 15 weeks, 26 weeks or, in some cases, 52 weeks.

Sick leave salary continuance plans have a range in level of benefit. Benefit levels can range from 57% to 100% of regular salary, up to a specified plan maximum. There is tremendous variance in non-work-related coverage for employees.

The employer may administer the sick leave plans in-house through human resources or occupational health or they may have an external third-party administrator who will administer the plan for them. External third-party administrators usually have specific forms for the collection of

Table 8.1 Example of a sick leave plan

Length of service (years)	Salary level while disabled (%)	Duration (weeks)
<1	100	2
	57	2–15
1–2	100	3
	57	3–15
2–3	100	4
	57	4–15
3–4	100	5
	57	5–15
4–5	100	6
	57	6–15
etc.	etc.	etc.

adequate information to administer the disability plan such as attending physicians' statements which need to be completed to apply and qualify for the company sick leave benefit. The programmes are based on sufficient objective medical documentation to support the absence. Third-party administrators generally use a solid DM framework to adjudicate and manage claims and to help employees obtain appropriate care and ultimately return to work (RTW). Third-party administrators are guided by company policies in their adjudication and management of claims. They use a variety of funding mechanisms to cover the cost of administering the claims; they usually do not issue the payment to the employee as this remains the employer's responsibility. This is an advantage to the employer as it keeps the employer's name in front of the employee even when they are absent on disability.

Sick leave plans have a variety of designs. Public sector organizations commonly have sick leave accumulation plans; these may also be called salary continuance. The level of benefit could be tied to years of service and there is often a reaccumulation element if days are used for sickness.

An example of such a plan is shown in Table 8.1. Sick leave plan eligibility is governed by employer policies, collective agreements and third-party agreements.

Short-term disability

Alternatively, the employer may have an insured short-term disability (STD) programme (these are also called weekly indemnity plans in some settings). These plans are negotiated with an insurer to administer the claims against a specific insurance company policy. Again, the level of benefit varies greatly, ranging from 57% to 100% of pre-illness income up to specified maximums. Waiting periods will be in place and vary by employer. Generally, these policies are established on a paid claims plus administration plus insurance company charges basis. It is a means of employers spreading the cost of disabilities over a longer period of time.

For example, if the employer will have Can$90 000 in claims in any given year, the insurer will put on 20–35% on top of this to cover their internal insurance charges and projections, bringing the cost of the programme to approximately Can$120 000. Therefore, the employer will pay Can$10 000 a month to the insurer to cover the cost of the claims over the year. The cost may be 100% paid by the employer, or employees may share the cost of the premiums. In some cases an employee's trade union may sponsor a disability plan for members. The union would negotiate with an insurer for this coverage and bill it back to their members. Generally, insurers use the last three years of experience to set the rates for the current year. There are several funding and insurance options available to employers who choose to use this method of coverage. The insurer will often issue the cheque to the employee in these arrangements.

There are specific claim submission requirements including immediate notification of the workplace to indicate absence; this is generally directed to the immediate supervisor and allows for planning of adequate coverage at the workplace to accomplish production. If the absence is expected to exceed three to five days (depending on the plan) an 'Attending Physician's Statement', which includes provision of sufficient objective medical information to support the disability, would be filed with the insurer for claim initiation.

Following the sick leave or STD phase the employer may or may not have a long-term disability plan.

Long-term disability

Long-term disability (LTD) plans vary greatly and may be insured or self-funded by the employer. The premiums may be paid by the employer, the employee or through a cost-splitting arrangement. Longterm disability plans will have a 'qualifying or elimination period' but generally this does not commence until after 17 weeks, 26 weeks or, in rare circumstances, 52 weeks. The plan designs can be varied and a range of benefit levels can be available up to 100% of income replacement with specific maximums. Most LTD plans are run through an insured arrangement due to the financial liabilities associated with long-term disabilities.

There is a specific application process for LTD which includes information from the employer, the employee and the treating physician(s) and specialist(s). This process can be a lengthy one and employees are encouraged to start the paperwork at least four to six weeks before the LTD phase of their disability starts.

With LTD benefits which are governed by an insurance company contract, DM practitioners should have a level of familiarity with the insurance company policy that controls the plan in their workplaces. There are many variations of funding and many options for plan design. One of the common plan designs is 60% of gross income up to a specified maximum for two years 'own occupation' then the definition may change to 'any occupation'. 'Own occupation' is defined as being unable to perform the 'essential duties' of their own pre-disability position. 'Any occupation' is defined as being unable to perform 'any' occupation that is reasonable by way of education, training and experience.

Individuals may be eligible for other income from other sources. However, the majority of LTD plans reduce these benefits from the amount they pay out to the employee while absent with a disability. An example of this offset is the CPP where government benefits are a direct reduction from the LTD payment. An example of the LTD benefit is Can$1000 and as the CPP is approved at Can$400 per month the LTD benefit would be reduced to Can$600. Most LTD policies make the application for CPP mandatory. Workers' compensation is another example. If the employee is receiving benefits from workers' compensation these will directly reduce the amount of LTD paid to that employee. There are also systems in place to prevent employees from making more income while on disability than they could have made while at work.

Some LTD policies include a mandatory rehabilitation provision where the employee is offered an opportunity to enter a rehabilitation programme and he or she has an obligation to participate. The consequence of not participating in a suitable LTD rehabilitation plan is the termination of benefits.

Long-term disability plans also usually include an 'all-source maximum' where the employee can only earn up to a specified maximum while on LTD. A common 'all-source maximum' is 85%. This is useful in the RTW phase of a disability as it protects the earnings level of employees while they try to transition back to the workplace without interfering with the rehabilitation process.

Long-term disability plans may have exclusions concerning a pre-existing condition. If the employee has such a condition that he or she came to the employer with, they may be excluded from the LTD insurance plan.

Once the LTD coverage period is over the employee may rely on government-sponsored benefits if they are still disabled and unable to return to work.

Claim submission evaluation

The non-occupational claims submission evaluation process will have the following components:

- receipt and review of the claim
- sufficient medical evidence to support the absence
- establishment of the employee status/eligibility for benefits under the plan
- participation in appropriate treatment
- review of the plan documents for any limitations in coverage; for example, conditions such as a result of pursuit of cosmetic surgery (that is not medically necessary), war, riot, self-inflicted injury and work-related absences may be excluded

- other exclusions as in the policy, contract or collective agreement
- pre-existing conditions may not be covered under some policies.

If there are no benefits available from the employer, the employee will be reliant on the government plans that they may qualify for given their eligibility and disability circumstances.

Recurrences

A recurrence is a situation where an employee has returned to employment following an absence and subsequently suffers a relapse or an aggravation of the original injury or illness. There is a wide variety of policy deviations on this issue. However, usually if the employee returns to work and becomes unable to work due to the same disability within two weeks (sometimes four weeks), as defined by the company or insurance company policy, he or she will go back onto the initial claim. If the absence is due to a completely different reason it will start a new claim.

It should also be noted that in some countries with universal disability schemes it does not matter if the disability is work-related or not – the application for benefits is the same.

Occupational

The main priority following a work-related accident is the employee. The first step is to determine if the employee requires first aid or external medical care.

FIRST AID

Specific regulations exist to ensure that employers have first aid available for employees if an injury should occur. The first aid station needs to have adequate emergency medical supplies. The workplace must have trained first aiders who can render first aid if required. Every time first aid is given it must be documented with details of the incident and the treatment provided.

EXTERNAL MEDICAL TREATMENT

If employees require treatment beyond first aid and are proceeding to external medical treatment they should be sent with a functional abilities evaluation form for immediate completion and return to the workplace. The form should be designed specifically around your workplace environment to ensure that the information received is unique to your workplace and employee needs. The healthcare provider should complete this and send it with the employee back to the workplace. The information surrounding the condition and the capabilities should be completed. This information should be used for the immediate offer of RTW (regular or modified) and for completion of the required notification to the Workers' Compensation Board or Insurer.

ACCIDENT INVESTIGATION: OCCUPATIONAL

An accident investigation should be performed immediately following a work-related incident or accident. It is important to do this promptly so that facts are not forgotten or the scene altered prior to an investigation. Accident investigations should include the supervisor, the injured employee, witnesses and, when applicable, the Joint Health and Safety Committee and/or the Union.

All accidents, no matter how apparently minor, should be investigated. The investigation is an investment in safety which pays direct dividends by helping to prevent future accidents. As discussed in Wilson and McCutcheon (2003), 'the importance of incident investigation can not be overstated. The basic causes have to be determined in order to provide the key solutions that will prevent future accidents'.

Components of a good accident investigation include:

- investigating the accident scene promptly
- completing the proper investigation reports in detail without delay to determine the root cause
- following-up to make sure appropriate corrective action has been taken
- accident reports, all of which should be reviewed at the monthly Joint Health and Safety Committee meetings
- determining if safety rules need to be modified and company procedures updated to prevent further accidents
- safety investigation findings and corrective actions at management meetings.

The investigation should always ensure that the root cause is uncovered. The process of root-cause analysis will allow for the discovery of the very basic factors that caused the accident. Root-cause identification requires critical analysis of the incident and the inquisitive method of asking why. At least three levels of exploration should be undertaken to discover the root causes. Take, for example, a male employee who gets a chemical splash in his eyes. The initial accident investigation (under corrective actions) indicates 'employee should use protective eyewear when pouring chemicals'. However, when we dig deeper we discover that the employee was newly hired, he had not received a full orientation, the chemical did not have a posting indicating that safety eyewear was required, and there was no eyewear close to the chemical pouring area. This example, albeit simple, shows how the root-cause analysis uncovered the necessity of better orientation training, workplace signage and improved availability of personal protective equipment.

A review of all accidents should be included in weekly management meetings. Elevating the focus on accidents – not only the reporting of the accident but also the correction of the root cause – puts accountability on the manager and supervisors to ensure that the incident does not occur again. Leadership within an organization sets the direction, aligns the staff, and provides motivation and inspiration to energize people into working safely. A visible commitment to a safe working environment is essential for the prevention of accidents.

CLAIM SUBMISSION: REPORTING OBLIGATIONS

Information collected during the accident/incident investigation should be used for the completion of the initial accident report. The employer should not attempt to diagnosis the injury on the initial submission. For example, avoid statements such as 'he sprained his ankle'. Employers should only report the details they know.

It is good practice to have a simple instruction sheet available for employees so that they can understand the steps in the workers' compensation process. The instruction sheet should include information on the process and who to contact at each step. This provides clarity around roles and responsibilities, and reduces the uncertainty following an accident.

In submitting information to the Workers' Compensation Board or Insurer, employers are guided by the workers' compensation legislation in their country and ultimately their province or state. Predominantly the responsibility exists to notify as soon as possible after acquiring knowledge of the accident if the accident required external healthcare intervention or modification of work. There are specific timelines in many jurisdictions often requiring notice within three days. There is a penalty ranging from Can$250 to Can$25 000 for non-submission or late filing of claims.

Many jurisdictions have specific forms that need to be completed to initiate the claim. At a minimum the following details must be conveyed:

- occurrence and nature of the accident
- time of occurrence
- name and address of the employee
- place where the accident occurred
- name and address of the healthcare provider attending the injured employee
- any details respecting the accident.

If a company finds that a claim is questionable, it has the opportunity to say so on the form and attach a letter of explanation. In order for a claim to be accepted by the Workers' Compensation Board or Insurer, a worker must have sustained 'a personal injury or accident arising out of and occurring in the course of employment'. In the adjudication of the claim the Workers' Compensation Board or Insurer will ensure that the following exist:

- an accident
- personal injury
- proof of accident
- the accident must arise out of and occur in the course of employment
- the disability must be compatible with the claimed accident.

The workers' compensation system will look for the following indicators to determine admissibility of a claim.

Strenuous activity

If the worker was involved in very strenuous work, a causal relationship is more likely than if the worker was involved in very light work. However, strenuous work in and of itself is not an indicator of a work relationship and there is usually some causative circumstance which operates in concert with the strenuous work.

Recent changes

If there have been recent changes in the worker's job, or in the manner in which the duties are to be carried out, and the worker experiences an onset of disability within a reasonable time of this change, then this suggests a strong causal relationship. For example, 'strenuous work' is a cause if it is new to the specific workers.

Immediate reporting

If a worker advises the employer shortly after a change in duties that he or she is experiencing a disability, this assists in establishing a causal relationship.

Immediate medical attention

This supports a relationship. The board will only compensate for medically supported disability. If the worker did not seek medical attention then no claim will be established.

Repetitive movement

If the job involves repetitive lifting, bending, twisting, etc., even in the absence of a specific incident, a causal relationship may be considered.

Awkward movement

If the worker's job requires him or her to move in an awkward manner, this will assist in the establishment of the causal relationship.

Requirement for lost time

If modified work is offered by the employer immediately, it decreases the chances of a lost-time claim. The Workers' Compensation Board or Insurer will look at the employee's capabilities versus the job requirements to determine how reasonable the offer is. If the offer is reasonable, the employee has the obligation to attend work and perform the modified duties (WSIB 2004).

Generally, in most of the workers' compensation systems the benefit of the doubt goes to the worker if there is a question about the probability of the accident or the lost time. It is of the utmost importance that all details and information relevant to the claim be included with the initial submission. The employer should keep a copy of the initial submission on file.

PRE-EXISTING CONDITIONS

In most workers' compensation systems, if the employee has a pre-existing condition, there may be an opportunity for cost-sharing on the claim. This would include situations where the employee has previous claims or previous personal conditions that may influence the amount of time off. Employers can apply for cost relief to the respective Workers' Compensation Board.

Recurrences

In the workers' compensation system the claim may be reopened at any time if evidence substantiates a relationship between the current condition and the original claim. The claims adjudicator will require factual information to make a decision regarding continuing entitlement on a claim. The Workers' Compensation Board reviews the prior injury and new complaints to verify that the same, or a closely related, diagnosis has been established. The two key elements are continuity of medical treatment and continuity of complaints.

Each Workers' Compensation Board or Insurer has specific forms for this reason; the initial 'report of accident' form should not be used here. A letter should be used or recurrence forms, providing the full particulars of the employee's symptoms, facts surrounding the onset of symptoms, the original claim number, the date of original injury, and the name and address of the employer (if different from the current employer). The letter should indicate why the new symptoms should be allocated to the old claim number.

The cost impact should be evaluated prior to submitting a claim for recurrence in order to assess the possibility of avoiding high reserves that may be detrimental to premium rates or experience rating adjustments.

POTENTIAL OFFSETS OF LIABILITIES: THIRD-PARTY CLAIMS

In some circumstances there may be an opportunity to offset the claim costs by allocating the claim to a third party. This would be applicable if the third party had caused the accident. An example of this would be if an employee was hit by a truck driven by XYZ Co., i.e. someone other than the employer's employee. The company could apply to the Workers' Compensation Board to have the costs transferred to XYZ Co. The company should file the appropriate documentation and copy it to the legal department at the Workers' Compensation Board or Insurer.

CONCLUSION

Claims initiation is the first step in establishing a disability claim. Occupational and non-occupational submission practices vary but both require substantive medical evidence to support the disability and requirement for lost time.

REFERENCES

Shannon H, Lowe G 2002 How many injured workers do not file claims for workers' compensation benefits? American Journal of Industrial Medicine 42:467–473

Wilson L, McCutcheon D 2003 Industrial Safety and Risk Management. The University of Alberta Press, Edmonton, Alberta

Workplace Safety and Insurance Board 2004 Operational Policy Manual. WSIB Publication, Toronto

Chapter 9

Claim and case management

LEARNING OBJECTIVES

■ Understand the claim and case management processes
■ Know how to monitor and manage cases
■ Be aware of external resources and different speciality interventions
■ Recognize the importance of appropriate case management methods
■ Understand the potential impact of good case management

INTRODUCTION

Case management is an important component of the disability management (DM) programme. Case management provides the ongoing connection between all parties, thereby becoming the communication link between the disabled employee, the workplace and the healthcare providers during absence and recovery. Contact should be frequent and should contain important messages of genuine concern for the employee, expectations that the employee will comply with company policies, participate in appropriate treatment and that there is a workplace commitment to return the employee to work within their capabilities.

Claims management refers to the paper processing of the claim and the documentation required to administer the claim decisions on entitlement. Claims management is the first step in establishing any entitlement to benefits and the comparison of the medical documentation to the plan or policy description. This term is frequently used by insurance companies in their role as the administrators of the disability insurance company policy. It also extends to the point in the claim where supplemental medical information is received and where a determination needs to be made as to whether the medical documentation is within the parameters of the policy or plan documentation.

Case management consists of monitoring the progression of healthcare and recovery from the time the claim is initiated until return to regular work. Case management has had many terms applied to it over the years, such as 'disease management', 'rehabilitation management' and 'medical case management'. However, the definition can be summarized as 'the coordination of services to assist an individual back to function and ultimately in all but terminal cases back into the workforce'. Case management, when handled carefully and systematically, helps disabled employees receive high-quality care that is appropriate and cost-effective. It applies theories of managed care so that employees progress smoothly from one stage of recovery to the next until they are at maximum function. Depending on the circumstances it can involve many members of the DM team.

CLAIM MANAGEMENT

The paper part of the process has a few key elements including claim receipt, eligibility determination, contract parameter review, sufficient medical documentation and appeals.

CLAIM RECEIPT

Once the paperwork has been submitted it is usually:

- stamped
- registered as received
- forwarded to adjudication
- assigned a claim number.

This is the first step in the administrative process in the claim cycle.

ELIGIBILITY

Determination of eligibility is in accordance with workers' compensation legislation definitions, company policy or insurance company contract provisions. Not every employee, in every company in every situation, is covered. The following are some of the essential eligibility considerations that are reviewed:

Occupational eligibility

This type of eligibility comprises:

- employee of company
- work-related incident
- medical aid or lost time.

Non-occupational eligibility

This type of eligibility comprises:

- employee of company
- employee with coverage, e.g. full-time, meets qualification hours or waiting period

Figure 9.1 Claim management flowchart.

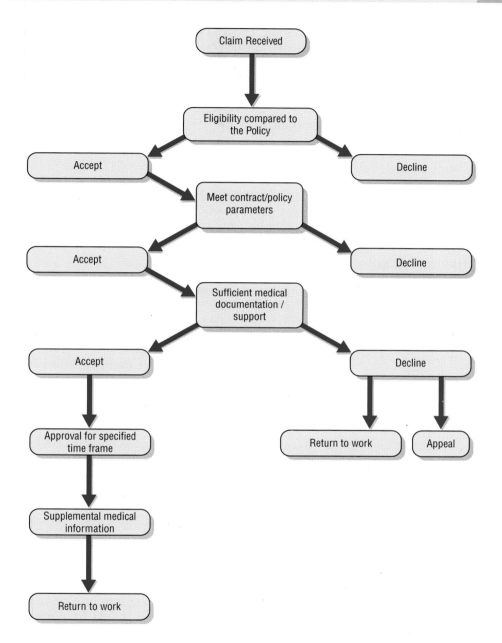

- policy date (disability occurred following the effective date of policy)
- covered employee (may have opted out of flex benefit plan).

CONTRACT OR POLICY PARAMETERS

All disability plans are governed by either legislation, policy or plan documents. There may be specific exclusions that exist in these documents. For example, 'stress' is specifically excluded from most workers' compensation legislation unless it is post-traumatic in origin. Another example is in the fact that many non-occupational plans exclude cosmetic surgery if it is not required for medical reasons. If someone chooses to have a face-lift and requires two weeks off to heal they would not be granted disability coverage for that time off. Some of the common contract or policy parameters include:

- limitations
- exclusions, e.g. war, riot, cosmetic surgery (when not medically necessary), working for another employer, participation in the armed forces or incarceration
- pre-existing conditions (in some policies)
- other insurance or policy clauses.

SUFFICIENT MEDICAL DOCUMENTATION

Medical documentation will be reviewed to determine if it is sufficient to disable the employee from the performance of their occupation; not all medical conditions are disabling in nature. It is important that initial forms are completed appropriately and fully to prevent needless denials. Payment is usually approved for a specific time then additional medical documentation will be required and reviewed to determine ongoing entitlement to benefits.

APPEAL

If a claim is denied the employee can appeal with additional medical information but such information must be new and unreviewed to substantiate the claim.

Case management

Once a claim is approved case management can commence, which should only be conducted by those with the appropriate skills, capabilities and knowledge. Case management is a different skill from return to work (RTW) planning as it involves interacting with the employee, the workplace and the healthcare community to ensure prompt and appropriate care. Disability management practitioners should have expertise and training in case management and healthcare, and they should perform these functions within a framework of DM principles and methods, ethical practice, laws and regulations, understanding of the business environment and current best practices in DM.

PROACTIVE INTERVENTIONS

Communication is the primary principle that case management is based on and it is used to ensure that the employee is aware of the options available right from the start of the disability. As discussed in McIntyre (2003), numerous studies have demonstrated that well-informed and fully involved patients make better use of treatment and get better results. Similarly, the collaborative process of case management promotes patient advocacy and enhances communication among patients, families, physicians and the employer. Properly implemented case management is an ongoing, proactive process that assesses, plans, implements, coordinates, monitors and evaluates available resources to ensure that the patient receives the most cost-effective and highest quality care needed to achieve the best possible outcome.

Preventing lost time is the first and most important strategy. In work-related cases, once the accident has been reported, the investigation report completed and healthcare intervention obtained, if necessary, possibilities to prevent lost time can be reviewed. If employees are capable of performing some duties, every effort should be made to avoid lost time. If employees require healthcare treatment they should have a functional abilities form that can guide the initial placement. In non-work-related conditions it is important to be aware of the current healthcare status (either physical or psychological) and be equally as prepared to facilitate return to work as soon as possible.

In cases where the employee requires lost time from work contact, intervals will be determined by the severity of the condition and case management activities guided by the type of claim. As discussed in Bigos et al (1989), the longer an employee is off work the less likely it is that they will ever return. Only 50% of employees ever return to work if disabled for longer than six months; only 10–15% of employees return to work if off work for longer than one year.

In reviewing cases we can categorize them into three major types of claims, which all demand different intervention strategies.

The first type is the short-duration absence, where the individual has a well-defined acute episode. These cases are short and employees return to work easily at the end of the episode. An example of this would be a simple virus such as the flu; it has a defined period of illness and the individual comes back to work well and ready to function fully.

The second type is where employees with an illness, disease or injuries will benefit from interventions. This group is where case management strategies need to be implemented to ensure they receive appropriate care and can transition back to work. They may need assistance in the healthcare system or they may need reinforcement that return to work is the primary objective.

The third type is where the employee has a terminal or debilitating disease that may preclude them from return to work. The primary need of this group is assistance in finding the best care possible, including services in the community.

In order to determine the type of absence there are key steps that the DM practitioner will follow, as detailed below.

Identification and referral

Identification involves the claim submission process. This creates the awareness that an individual is in fact claiming a disability. Eligibility will be determined based on the disability benefit parameters, either the internal company policy, the insurance company policy or the workers' compensation legislation. Then the DM practitioner reviews the case to determine which claims may require case management interventions. This process can be compared to a triage process where individuals are put in groups based on the severity or seriousness of their needs. Most Type One claims do not require intervention beyond the initial assessment.

Information collection

The next step is to gather relevant data on the case. This includes an assessment of the physical or psychological status of the employee, a determination of the current health status and treatment, identification of any resource needs, an identification of any barriers to treatment and an estimate of the employee's RTW timeline. The DM practitioner will evaluate all factors that may influence the case outcome including workplace factors and external factors. The information collection will include reviews of the job description and job demands analysis, as well as identification of any barriers that may prevent early and safe return to work.

Planning

The DM practitioner then determines if case management is appropriate. The practitioner (or case manager) will:

- maintain contact with the injured or ill employee, workplace parties and service providers
- assess the medical, psychological and external factors influencing the disability
- identify 'red flags' or barriers
- review the care and the response to treatment
- facilitate care and independent assessments (as required)
- review essential duties of the job and perform the match with the employee's capabilities
- facilitate RTW
- develop appropriate RTW plans and monitor for success
- work conditioning
- explore rehabilitation alternatives if a transition to a regular job is not feasible
- collect data to demonstrate the cost-effectiveness of DM interventions.

Maintain contact with the injured or ill employee, workplace parties and service providers

The role of the employee with the disability is very much an active role. The employee should be encouraged to actively pursue appropriate healthcare and return to work as soon as possible.

If the workplace has a DM practitioner, this individual's role is as the key coordinator of communication with all relevant parties. One role is to make sure the employee is focusing on RTW. It is also essential to coordinate the healthcare service providers to ensure that the employee is receiving the best possible healthcare to help his or her recovery. Case management is a goal-directed intervention process. Information is gathered and evaluated to determine the needs of the employee. It looks at all the key variables that can influence lost time and any barriers to return to work. The DM practitioner facilitates the planning of care and the selection of resources. It is necessary to establish a plan that will lead to the reintroduction of the worker to the workplace.

Workplace representatives, such as unions, may also have a role in the DM programme, particularly when it is time for the employee to return to work. It is positive to have these representatives communicating the objectives and the positive benefits of the programme.

Assess the medical, psychological and external factors influencing the disability

Lowery (2002) discusses some of the components in case management, early identification and prevention of complications, the removal of medical and psychological barriers to recovery, and assistance with timely return to work. The interventions can include any number of areas of assistance. It could be facilitating an appointment with a specialist, involving appropriate resources, referring to a second opinion, assistance in obtaining healthcare interventions, education for the employee or the physician on treatment options, identification of current capabilities, and evaluating the workplace for modified work or work-modification opportunities. The DM practitioner can assist the absent employee to navigate through the healthcare process. The practitioner has probably helped many disabled employees through the process whereas the employee has only had the disability once, making this resource invaluable.

The best overall approach is to focus on the functional capacity of the individual not the cure. It is important that the RTW expectation is clear. A clear DM action plan should be documented and regularly updated. Documentation is vital to effective case management as it helps provide:

- a profile of the claim status and the services required
- a good communication tool among parties
- a basis for planning recovery.

It is important to mention that all disability files should be dealt with in a confidential manner.

Identify 'red flags' or barriers

Some of the indicators that the case may be prolonged or not progressing according to the case management plan may include:

- a vague, multiple-diagnosis or poorly outlined treatment plan
- absence problem prior to disability
- pending litigation
- workers' compensation case with lost time
- duration of disability initially projected as longer than six weeks

- presence of performance or discipline problems
- lack of supportive clinical tests to support the condition
- delays in the RTW date
- 'doctor shopping'
- non-compliance with the treatment plan.

Review the care and the response to treatment

The element of proactive intervention-focused care management is the core of any case management programme. Services may be external or internal and include:

- coordinating and monitoring medical and rehabilitation services
- developing a recovery plan and case-coordination activities among the employee and healthcare providers
- developing transitional work plans with the employee, management, treating healthcare providers, and employee representatives (when necessary)
- coordinating of Independent Medical Examinations (IMEs) and Functional Abilities Evaluations (FAEs)
- reviewing job analysis information to understand the type of work the employee is able to perform
- arranging vocational assessments to evaluate transferable skills.

Case management is performed on a multidisciplinary platform collaborating with all essential parties to ensure the best outcome. The case manager is the liaison in the system to solve the problems faced by workers and employers in the disability process. Case management may include assessing, planning, implementing, coordinating, monitoring and evaluating the services available to meet individual health needs and promote early and safe return to work.

Facilitate care and independent assessments

Use of preferred providers

In an effort to ensure that employees can receive appropriate care, many employers and third-party administrators have negotiated strategic alliance arrangements with preferred providers. A preferred provider can be in any discipline from physiotherapy to psychological counselling. The intent is to achieve preferred access with service expectations and measured results.

One of the important elements when selecting preferred providers is to ensure that they support the case management and early and safe RTW philosophy. If you align with a provider who is not supportive of this philosophy it can be a recipe for disaster. An example of how these relationships can go wrong would be if there is a physiotherapy clinic in town which the workplace has toured and selected to negotiate with to take their employees on a prompt basis. The physiotherapy clinic toured the workplace and observed the jobs, assisted in some on-site ergonomics training to help all the employees perform the work more effectively and they became familiar with the modified work that may be available. Arrangements were then made to have the physiotherapy clinic treat a few employees. The physiotherapist, instead of adopting the employer's early and safe RTW attitude, proceeded to be overly sympathetic to the employees. The physiotherapist supported employee concerns during discussions that the jobs were repetitive, difficult in nature, and not a job she would like to perform. She did not encourage the employees to try new techniques to make the job easier to perform, did not support early return to work and ended up prolonging lost time and extending treatment programmes due to the lack of work conditioning involvement in the programme. This is an example that emphasizes the necessity of having providers that not only tour the workplace but understand the early and safe RTW philosophy.

Role of IMEs and FAEs

If the employee's condition is complex, approaching or exceeding the initial medical prognosis or the standard disability duration guidelines, or if it requires a second opinion, then the potential of using an IME or FAE should be reviewed. As discussed in Knoblauch and Strasser (2002) an independent assessment can be defined as a comprehensive evaluation of a health-related issue by a healthcare professional who has no interest in and agrees not to subsequently treat the involved employee.

An IME is an examination performed by a medical practitioner other than the employee's own personal physician. It is important to ensure that the qualifications of the independent examiner are in the specific area of expertise related to the 'concern'. IME providers should be evaluated to ensure that they are in the right specialty, they have appropriate credentials, expertise and experience, a good reputation, no biases and are prepared to have a suitable turn-around time. A specialized IME may be indicated when:

- the employee is not progressing and a second opinion may be useful
- the ongoing disability is prolonged and without apparent resolution
- there is a need to clarify the initial and/or longterm ability to return to work
- there is serious doubt that the initial injury or ongoing disability is related to the injury or accident.

A copy of the employee's job description detailing specific physical demands, if available, and modified work alternatives should be sent to the treating physician prior to the appointment.

An FAE is an objective method of assessing physical abilities and limitations. These are performed by specialized healthcare personnel, usually physiotherapists, occupational therapists or kinesiologists. They can measure physical tolerances and capabilities, and they can also be used to assist in the identification of treatment options that may improve outcomes.

In work-related cases the employee is legally obliged to participate in an IME or FAE. If the employee does not comply they should be contacted to determine the reason for the refusal. If the reason is not acceptable, a workers' compensation appeal should be initiated and the employee notified they are in breach of the Act (WSIB 2004a,b) and at risk of losing benefits. Workers' compensation should be notified of the refusal and the circumstances.

In non-work-related cases the employee may be obliged to attend an IME or FAE depending on the wording of the policies and/or insurance company contract.

The goal of an IME or FAE is to resolve the issues and obtain a credible medical opinion that will be accepted by the Workers' Compensation Board, Insurer or third-party administrator, the employee and the employee's physician. It is important that a specialist in the relevant area of disability conduct the IME. The qualifications of the physician and his or her ability to evaluate a case impartially should be emphasized and detailed.

The IME physician should be provided with the following information:

- a covering letter that states the specific questions on the issues to be resolved
- employee information
- a chronological outline of the history of the case
- documentation that details how the accident occurred and what the initial injuries were
- a copy of the workers' compensation claim file (if available)
- any other information available that can be released, e.g. RTW slips
- pre-injury job description and physical demands analysis
- a list of questions that need to be answered.

Following an IME or FAE the case manager's role is to review the capabilities and limitations information obtained and compare it to the job demands. The process simply takes the employee's abilities and compares them to the job demands. If these abilities do not tally with the employee's own occupation the information can then be used to see if they match an alternative job in the company.

Review essential duties of the job and perform the match with the employee's capabilities

When the employee has the capabilities to transition back to work the essential duties of the job can be matched to the employee's capabilities. The process of job matching will ensure there is a reduced risk of re-injury in the placement.

Facilitate return to work

Return to work can be as simple as an employee returning to full function in the workforce based on recovery and capabilities. It is important that RTW dates are communicated promptly to the supervisor or manager to allow for appropriate scheduling of the workforce.

Develop appropriate return-to-work plans and monitor for success

When an employee requires transitional or modified work a clear RTW plan should be established based on the capability of the employee to perform the essential duties of the job. The progress back to regular duties should be monitored both from the medical and the job site point of view.

Work conditioning

Employees who have become disabled often become physically 'deconditioned' if they are off work for extended periods. The activities of work may involve using muscles that have not been used during the absence. Work-conditioning programmes are often an extension of the physiotherapy programme and assist in trying to improve the employee's physical tolerance to job-related activities. Work conditioning can be done at the physiotherapy clinic or on-site at the workplace through a gradual build-up of activities. If work conditioning is carried out at the clinic it is good practice to have work simulation equipment available or even a replica of the workplace task or production line to make the work conditioning as relevant and specific as possible.

Explore rehabilitation alternatives if a transition to a regular job is not feasible

In some cases the employee will not be able to return to work to their previous job or maybe not even to the same workplace. It is important to explore rehabilitation alternatives when this occurs. This assessment should include components such as personal factors, transferable skills, aptitude testing, interest testing, vocational factors, medical factors, psychosocial factors, educational factors and financial factors.

Collect data to demonstrate the cost–effectiveness of disability management interventions

The DM practitioner will be collecting overall statistical data to support the programme and demonstrate their cost-effectiveness and ability to meet targets and goals. However, on a case-by-case basis it is useful to demonstrate the impact of the interventions. These can be tracked by projecting the cost of the claim without interventions and documenting the cost of the claim with the interventions.

CONCLUSION

Once the case management goals have been achieved the case can be closed. The claim and case management process is an important component in the DM programme. It provides the intervention steps from the time the employee goes off work to the time the individual is ready to return. Interventions in this segment of the claim can assist in reducing the duration of the claims.

REFERENCES

Bigos S J, Spengler D M, Martin N A 1989 Low back pain in industry: a retrospective study. Spine 11:252–256

Knoblauch D J, Strasser P B 2002 Managing employee health problems – optimal use of independent medical evaluations. American Association of Occupational Health Nurses Journal 50(12):549–552

Lowery S 2002 Case management: you really do get what you pay for. Business and Health Institute, 3 October, 1–6

McIntyre K L A 2003 Managing large claims down to size. Business and Health, 1 August, p 21

Workplace Safety and Insurance Board 2004a Operational Policy. Ontario (http://www.wsib.on.ca)

Workplace Safety and Insurance Board 2004b The Workplace Safety and Insurance Act. Ontario http://www.wsib.on.ca

Chapter 10

Return to work

LEARNING OBJECTIVES

- To be able to differentiate between return-to-work levels of complexity
- Understand the role of key indicators in return to work
- Understand the importance of bridging the gap between recovery and return to work

---

INTRODUCTION

Even though disability management (DM) reaches far beyond this activity alone, return to work (RTW) remains the most visible activity of most DM programmes. It certainly is the area in which many success stories are written. However, RTW is not a one-dimensional process. In fact it is multidimensional, ranging from the level of the simplest interventions to the most complex interventions.

SIMPLE RETURN TO WORK

In many or most cases very little assistance is required to return someone to work. Cases become more complex and difficult to resolve if action is not taken as soon as possible. It is quite possible that a RTW can be arranged without the assistance of a DM practitioner. If the attending physician is clear in identifying restrictions, and if these restrictions are minor in nature, the worker can supply the worksite with this information and a RTW can be arranged.

For example, a male worker sustains a severe splinter injury in the thumb of his non-dominant hand. He receives appropriate first aid followed by stitches at the emergency room. He sees his physician the next day who wants him to stay home until the wound heals. Three days later the physician says he can return to work if he keeps the hand dry and wears a protective glove. The worker passes this on to his foreman who checks with human resources. The accommodation can easily be arranged and the worker goes back without difficulty. This resolution presupposes that there is good communication between the worker, the physician and the employer. Most worksites have this level of communication; however, things become complicated when an insurer is involved.

If the case requires workers' compensation reporting, which it does in most jurisdictions, it is quite possible that the entire process will become prolonged. In some cases the paperwork for reporting this type of injury will not have been completed before the worker in this example has already returned to his job. Even if the employer is very quick to report this incident to the compensation provider it is quite possible that the provider may take days to weeks to adjudicate the acceptance of this claim. This period may be long enough for other problems, such as emotional frustration, to kick in, which in turn may prolong the length of the claim. This is precisely why DM practitioners focus on solutions between the worker and the employer to act before the insurer acts. It is not unheard of for an insurer to take weeks to make a decision such as this and there is no reason why the employer, worker and physician cannot agree to move faster. There is always the prospect that the insurer may deny a claim. However, the costs of dealing with this proactively will be much less if lost wages are kept to a minimum. In unionized worksites it is ideal for the union to be involved in RTW planning including a simple one such as this.

Slightly more complex cases

The factor that usually moves simple cases to a more complex status is length of recovery. If the injury is such that the person is going to be away from work for several weeks there are a number of key steps that should be taken in order to minimize the chance of complications occurring (Box 10.1).

Medium–complexity cases

Medium complexity cases are defined by the need for temporary accommodations such as modifications to the workplace or work schedule. It should be noted that these are changes to the worksite, not adjustments the worker has to make. It is often the worker who is asked to adjust when it is clearly the moral obligation and perhaps contractual and legislative obligation of the employer to make the adjustment (Box 10.2).

Complex cases

Complex cases are distinguished from the less complex in that the nature of the disability is very difficult to accommodate. This may be as a result of a very unpleasant injury or secondary issues such as emotional trauma being present (Box 10.3).

Long–term absence

Long-term absences bring a unique challenge. Frequently, these cases are referred to a DM practitioner when the two-year window is about to expire and the person is being moved from the 'own occupation' category to the

Box 10.1 Key steps to be taken to minimize the chances of complications occurring during a prolonged absence from work

1. The injured worker must receive immediate and excellent medical care. It is imperative that there are no delays at this stage. The worker, and the worker's family, need to know that no expense will be spared to ensure survival and care at this stage. Immediate first aid, medivac, etc., are critical at this stage.

2. Once the worker is in a stable condition, he or she needs to know that their needs and the needs of their family will be met. This is the stage where information about the organization's disability plan and the DM process can be provided. It is critical that this is carried out in a tactful manner and with the greatest discretion. Nevertheless it is very important that it happens early in the process so that the worker experiences no additional stress that may interfere with the recovery process.

3. The care of the worker is monitored. Any problems with benefits, treatment, family, etc., need to be addressed and resolved. It is critical that the employer stays in touch with the worker so that the worker's position as a key contributor to the employer's business is maintained. It is such a simple yet overlooked part of the process and it pays great dividends when the worker continues to feel part of the worksite rather than feeling as if he or she has been ignored or cast aside. This contact can be fostered by co-workers or union members as well as other organizational representatives contacting the worker.

4. The process of planning the RTW should begin. Information should be gathered from the physician, the employer and the worker regarding potential barriers to a successful RTW. Collective agreements or RTW policies should be reviewed regarding their provisions. Advance work at this stage can smooth the way for a problem-free RTW once the worker is cleared to do so.

5. Set the stage for RTW. Prepare the worker, co-workers, supervisors, etc., for the imminent RTW. It is imperative that everyone who may have contact with the worker is aware of the restrictions of the RTW. This knowledge must be constrained by confidentiality provisions but such information as can be shared will allow everyone to work together to ensure a successful outcome.

6. The RTW should be designed in such a manner that it eases the worker back into their pre-accident or pre-illness employment. With relatively simple cases the most that is required is a graduated RTW (GRTW). In many instances two mistakes are made. One is to predetermine the length of the GRTW and saying, for example, that it will be six weeks long. It is our opinion that the maximum initial expectation should be six weeks but in many instances this may be shorter. If a realistic period of six weeks is not likely then it should not be attempted. Understandably, employers become frustrated at long or unending GRTW arrangements. Failure of GRTW can usually be attributed to the RTW being attempted too early, before the worker is functionally ready. The second mistake is not being ready to address problems as they arise during the GRTW. It is common for the worker to encounter some difficulties during the process. It is better to be able to address these as they occur, at the worksite if at all possible, and keep the GRTW going rather than pull the worker out and start again at a later date. Every failed GRTW makes it that much more difficult for everyone involved to try again. The old axiom of 'failing to plan is planning to fail' really holds true here. The GRTW is a powerful tool and needs to be used with proper planning, evaluation and commitment to success. It is not something you do without thought or as a convenience or as an easy solution.

7. The RTW should be monitored and evaluated. Once it is over it is a good idea to ask the participants what worked well and what did not work. Identified issues may be addressed to the benefit of workers in need of this assistance in the future.

Box 10.2 Key steps in a medium-complexity RTW case

1., 2., 3. These steps are the same as in Box 10.1.
4. While the process of planning the RTW essentially remains the same there is a different goal. In simple RTW the goal is RTW without accommodation or at most a GRTW. With medium-complexity cases there is an acknowledgement or understanding at the outset that the nature of the injury or illness will require accommodation on the part of the employer. It is also understood that the accommodation is of a temporary nature as it is the goal of the intervention to return the worker to his regular job. It is very important to begin gathering information early in the process in order to avoid subsequent delays. There is no reason why this process has to wait until the worker has fully recovered. If not already on file, the employer should conduct a job demands analysis in order to quantify the tasks that the worker actually does as part of the employment. This will often vary from the job description which may be out of date or not accurately reflect the tasks completed. Even if the job description is current it is unlikely to contain the specific information that a job demands analysis provides. This detailed information then needs to be given to the medical professionals so that they can tailor treatment and make recommendations specific to the job demands analysis. The opinions of the medical professionals are then brought to the DM practitioner or RTW committee at the worksite who then make specific arrangements for the worker.
5. The accommodation needs to be monitored closely to ensure that it is meeting the needs of the worker and the workplace. Both parties need to be happy with the progress and if there are problems they should be addressed immediately. It is vital that regular and frequent contact be maintained with the worker and the worker's immediate supervisor. It is these individuals who will be able to provide the most accurate information. A daily log sheet can be introduced in cases where the worker needs to track specific activities.
6. With a medium-complexity case the accommodation is temporary. The goal of the accommodation is to return the workers to their regular jobs. Therefore this intervention is progressive and progress should be evaluated on this basis.
7. The outcomes should be evaluated and the case closed upon completion.

Box 10.3 Key steps in a complex RTW case

1., 2. These steps are the same as in Box 10.1 but it should be noted that the more serious the injury or illness the more important it is to 'do a good job' in the early stages. Everything that happens later in the process will be influenced by what happens at the outset.
3. While problems or complications do not only arise in more serious cases it is more likely that they will, given the length of recovery period.
4. Here it is acknowledged that a RTW will require extensive accommodations. In fact it may be unclear if it will be possible to accommodate the worker in a temporary manner. In this kind of case it may be wise to consider the possibility of the need for a permanent accommodation early in the process. Nevertheless, all attempts at accommodating the person in their original position should be vigorously pursued.

'any occupation', commonly referred to as the own occ./any occ. crisis. These are often people who have 'fallen off the radar' for a long time because they were initially deemed too seriously ill or too injured to work. Once the person is on long-term disability (LTD) benefits, many employers stop trying to assist the person. This is aided by the attitude of many unions who have requested a hands-off attitude once the person is on LTD. This request is fuelled by a misconception that once a person is on LTD they will probably never return to work and should be left alone to get on with their life as best they can – this is incorrect thinking. LTD benefits are not 100% income replacement. For many people on LTD their lifestyles slowly deteriorate into poverty and lose any focus on rehabilitative efforts.

Case study

A large mill had 76 workers on LTD. The mill had recently introduced a DM programme, which had strong support from senior administration and the union. The DM practitioners involved wanted to provide assistance to the workers on LTD. The union was of the opinion that these workers were ill, that they were entitled to LTD and should be left alone. After some further discussion it was decided that the workers should be the ones making the decision about whether to accept assistance or not, and the practitioners were given permission to contact the workers. To the surprise of many, most of the workers contacted stated that they wanted to get off LTD and return to work. The common response was that they were tired of trying to live on LTD and wanted to get on with their lives. Assistance, such as GRTW, job modifications, schedule changes, counselling, etc., was made available. Of the 76 workers, 38 returned to work within a year and the mill saved US$1.25 million. Given that the LTD plan was jointly funded the mill saved US$480000, which was shared among all workers (Hursh 1997). The workers also had their incomes restored and could get on with their lives.

Light–duty programmes

For many years light-duty programmes were seen as the programme of choice when assisting an injured worker to return to work. Some organizations went to great lengths to set up light-duty programmes but in most cases these were only arranged when needed. As a result of their 'one-off' nature they were subject to the vagaries of the economy, supervisor's good will and favouritism. Anecdotally, the industry is rife with stories of people who were not given light duties because they were not liked by the supervisor, or others who were allowed to stay at light duties for extended periods because they were well liked. In some cases, light duties would become permanent in that the worker would never go back to a regular job.

More commonly, light duties would often go on longer than planned. Frequently referred to as a graduated RTW (GRTW) these programmes are usually arranged for a period such as four to six weeks. If a person is not able to return to work at the end of this period, it is often extended. It is not uncommon for a GRTW to last for 12 weeks or longer and then still fail to return the person to their regular job. It is no wonder that employers and insurers began to look for other solutions. What on the surface looks like a good idea – light work until fully recovered – has one major Achilles' heal: the light-duty jobs usually have very little resemblance to the actual work that the employee will need to perform once back at the regular job. If this is the case, how then can this be therapeutic in any way? Historically it was not uncommon for the worker to be brought back and told to sit in the first aid room all day, or given some other menial work to do, such as unrolling and re-rolling bandages. Employees and their representatives (in unionized worksites) objected to this type of arrangement saying that it demeaned the individual and argued that work should be meaningful and productive. Employers also objected to this approach as making light duties available did nothing to help the person return to work and did not enhance productivity. In fact, some light-duty programmes were so attractive to employees that once accustomed to them they did not want to return to their regular work and delayed going back as long as possible. The more unpleasant the job they were returning to the more likely this would be.

In an effort to improve this situation some organizations set up more permanent light-duty programmes. Typically they tried to find a part of the operation that could be considered 'light' and then tried to reserve those for people coming back to work post-injury or -illness. This approach was also problematic as these jobs were usually obtained by more senior, usually older, workers who wanted those jobs to see them into retirement. Perhaps this is best illustrated with an example.

Case study

An open-pit mine with some 300 employees wanted a light-duty programme. They looked around their operation and decided that the electric motor rewinding shop was ideal. Workers coming back after injury could go and work in the shop for a length of time before going back to their regular jobs. The work in the shop was light and the shop was dry and heated. When it was first started the jobs in the shop were separate from the collective agreement and therefore not subject to seniority. Of course everyone in the mine wanted these jobs. The work was physically light, it was inside, it was dry and, compared to working outside in the mine, it was clean. Eventually, during bargaining, the jobs in the shop became part of the collective agreement and subject to seniority. In no time senior employees had bid on the jobs and the programme was gone.

Transitional work programmes

The idea of a transitional work programme (TWP) is discussed by Shrey (1995). He outlined a whole process of carrying out DM using transitional work. From that we have taken the notion of workers making the transition from being off work due to injury or illness back to their regular job through a transitional process. Also, unlike light duties or light-duty programmes, a TWP is a permanent feature of a worksite – it is negotiated, defined and stays in place at all times. Transitional work programmes allow injured workers to gradually and safely increase their work activities to full duty. In a TWP, the workers' tasks actually become part of their rehabilitation and help to facilitate the healing process. Employers also benefit. Transitional work programmes reduce the length of lost-time claims, reduce the need for replacement workers and give the employer an opportunity to assist the injured or ill employee to return to work at full duty.

A large, unionized shop in a major metropolitan area wanted to implement a TWP; they contracted with a DM provider to help them set it up. The DM provider met the employer and union and eventually a letter of understanding was signed which outlined the TWP. Then a group of occupational therapists were brought in to conduct job demands analysis, to assess the tasks and physical requirements of every position in the machine shop. While this was being completed it was noted that the machining process produced a large quantity of metal scraps. These were collected by an external firm and taken away. It was suggested that this process could possibly be used as part of the TWP. Each part of collecting and hauling the scraps away also underwent job demands analysis. Everything from sweeping, to wheel-barrowing, to driving equipment, etc., was analysed and catalogued. If possible, the jobs were broken down into individual components, such as weights, forces and repetitions. These descriptions were accompanied by photographs or videos of people doing those tasks. Then, when a worker was declared fit to begin work re-entry, the physician was supplied with a list of jobs and their physical requirements. If possible, the DMP met the physician and showed a video of the job. The physician was then able to tick off tasks that were appropriate (on a RTW form). The worker was then assigned the specific tasks from the TWP that were a proper fit with the physician's recommendations. For example, one worker may be assigned sweeping and another shovelling, depending on their physical restrictions and recovery needs. Each RTW is individually planned and monitored. By doing this, the tasks become part of the physical therapy. The DMP monitors the worker's progress and is in regular contact with the worker and others at the job site. The worker has new tasks assigned as appropriate. Should the worker encounter difficulties assistance, such as an occupational therapist, is brought to the worksite. Tasks are added from those available until the worker is back at the regular job. The process should not be started unless the medical treatment provider (MTP) is confident that the worker will be ready in six weeks. Remember that the purpose of the TWP is to help the workers make the transition back to their regular employment. If they are not ready, they should be allowed to recover for longer before the attempt is made. Many RTW programmes fail out of misguided, if well-meaning, attempts to get workers back to work too soon.

An added benefit of this TWP is that when there is no worker in need of the programme, the employer hires casual labour or students to do the work. The employer recycles the material to its own foundry; these savings are added to the TWP budget. This makes the programme almost completely self-financing even before the insurance cost savings are taken into account.

PERMANENT ACCOMMODATIONS

Much of the activity in DM is with people who have temporary disabilities. If someone has a permanent disability that prohibits them from doing their job – a permanent accommodation is needed. This is the field of ergonomists and occupational therapists. These professions have the skills necessary to assess the person, assess the work locations, assess the job tasks and make recommendations for appropriate accommodations. This is not usually within the training of a DM practitioner. However, DM practitioners need to be familiar with the appropriate resources in their community so that they can make the arrangements for such a process to take place.

Once a permanent accommodation has been made it is critical that there is regular follow-up with the person. There are many examples of people who were accommodated and then forgotten. While the person does have responsibility to advocate for their own needs, it is also the employer's responsibility to ensure that the individual continues to be accommodated. For example, if the accommodation involves computer hardware or software, regular upgrades will be required. If the person has a hearing aid, frequent maintenance and regular replacement will be required. In short, a permanent accommodation is not a one-off event. It is a lifelong process.

THE HIERARCHY OF RETURN TO WORK

Old hierarchy:

1. RTW – same employer, same job.
2. RTW – same employer, modified job.
3. RTW – same employer, new job.
4. RTW – new employer, new job.
5. Formal retraining.
6. Self-employment.

New hierarchy:

1. RTW – same employer, same job.
2. RTW – same employer, modified job, job accommodations.
3. RTW – same employer, new job.
4. Retraining and re-employment – same employer.
5. Retraining and job search.

The subtle but important difference between the two hierarchies is that all options, including physical accommodations, schedule changes, job task modifications, etc., and the acquisition of application of new skills in a new job, are exercised with the pre-injury or -illness employer. In the past, too many individuals have suffered long-term unemployment as a result of rehabilitation professionals engaging in social engineering experiments. Out of a misguided belief that everyone should have a better job, employment contracts were severed early in the process with catastrophic results when the person could not succeed at retraining or could not find new employment once the training was completed. Not everyone has the skills, motivation or desire to hold a more highly skilled or so called 'white-collar' job. The employment relationship should be severed only as a last resort and once all options have been exhausted.

Self-employment

For a while it was quite popular to encourage workers to leave their positions and take on some type of self-employment. Many attempts were made to purchase or set up small businesses such as shops, vending machine routes, launderettes, etc. Unfortunately, even the most well-motivated and experienced entrepreneurs fail at this. Self-employment is a daunting task not to be engaged in lightly. The work is hard, the hours long and the notion that 'when I'm self-employed I can set my own hours' is a lie. If this route of accommodation is to be taken it must be approached carefully, vigorously and with full due diligence. It should be stressed with the employee that this is a difficult undertaking fraught with risk and not the panacea that some people think it is. Caution, not urgency, is needed when considering self-employment, particularly when recovering from a disability.

Step-wise return-to-work outline

Minor injury or illness

1. Worker has an injury or becomes ill.
2. First aid attends, treats and files report.
3. Worker sees medical treatment practitioner (MTP).
4. Worker has no, or short period of, convalescence.
5. Worker returns to work – full-time, full duties.

More serious injury or illness

1. Worker has an injury or becomes ill.
2. First aid attends, treats and files report.
3. Worker is transported to hospital.
4. First aid, DM practitioner or designate accompanies worker to hospital.
5. DM practitioner stays with worker until stable, or until other support arrives.
6. DM practitioner speaks with worker or support person, reassures him or her, gives contact information and explains that contact will be taken up again as soon as appropriate.
7. DM practitioner ensures that all necessary paperwork is completed and that there is little likelihood of an interruption to benefits.
8. Worker receives excellent medical care.
9. DM practitioner is in touch with the worker and support network during the recovery process.
10. DM practitioner is in touch with the employer and union during the recovery process, and provides both of them with general information regarding recovery and eventual return to work.

11. DM practitioner is in contact with the MTP, ensuring that the MTP is aware of all the resources that are available to assist in the recovery of the worker.
12. Worker is referred to a rehabilitation clinic for treatment and activation therapy.
13. While the worker is in the clinic the DM practitioner is aware of the worker's progress and eventual RTW date. The practitioner is an external part of the clinic's treatment team.
14. As the worker nears the end of treatment at the clinic, the DM practitioner arranges for the worker to be admitted to the TWP.
15. Worker participates in TWP.
16. The DM practitioner ensures that the TWP unfolds as outlined above.
17. The DM practitioner ensures that the worker is familiar with the safety aspects of the TWP position(s).
18. After successful progression through the TWP, the worker returns to regular duties.
19. DM practitioner 'celebrates' success as appropriate with the worker and employer/union. It is critical that we celebrate our success not just revel in our failures.
20. DM practitioner ensures that the case is closed as appropriate and that all data for programme evaluation have been captured.

CONCLUSION

Arranging the RTW of an injured or ill worker is an important and sometimes complex activity. It is critical that the DM practitioner is proactive in this process in every respect, but most importantly in dealing with worker's, employer's and union's expectations. It should be made unapologetically clear that the goal of the process is the return of the person to their job, and that they will have the full support of the employer, union and workmates, but they will also have to do their part. It is vital to act early but not too early – timing is critical. Contact with the worker and the worker's support system is critical throughout the process. Workers must know that they are a valued member of the workforce, that they are missed, that they will be assisted back to work and welcomed once they get there. Paying attention to the person's psychosocial needs (support, self-esteem and mood) is as critical and perhaps more critical than addressing their physical needs. With the kind of proactive support outlined in this chapter worksites can arrange RTW programmes suitable to their individual needs and that will allow them to be more effective in accommodating workers with temporary and permanent disabilities in the worksite. This is an important undertaking not only for employers but for society as a whole. It is imperative that workers know that society acknowledges them to be valuable contributors to the fabric of our society and that they will not be discarded if they become ill or injured.

REFERENCES

Hursh N C 1997 Disability Management Program Graduates: Making a difference in the workplace. National Institute of Disability Management and Research (NIDMAR), Port Alberni, British Columbia

Shrey D E 1995 Disability management practice at the worksite: developing, implementing and evaluating transitional work programs. In: Shrey D E, Lacerte M (eds) Principles and Practices of Disability Management in Industry. GR Press, Winter Park, Florida

Chapter **11**

Rehabilitation

LEARNING OBJECTIVES

- Understand the development of medical and vocational rehabilitation
- Understand the difference between medical and vocational rehabilitation
- Understand the importance of recognizing and dealing with psychosocial issues in rehabilitation
- Recognize the value of comprehensive disability management

INTRODUCTION

Understanding current rehabilitation practices requires contextualization and a small historical excursion. Our current practices have evolved out of several key historical events. We will first examine the history of the development of medical rehabilitation.

MEDICAL REHABILITATION

Prior to World War I rehabilitation was unheard of. The simple truth was that people did not survive serious injuries, such as amputations, in any great numbers. If they did survive they were left as is and had to survive as well as they could, often in abject poverty. Advances in medical knowledge meant that more soldiers returned from World War I than had from previous wars and had to reintegrate into society. Many of these soldiers had physical and mental disabilities as a consequence of the war. Consequently, the first attempts were made to rehabilitate these individuals into 'normal' lifestyles. The emphasis was on physical disabilities. Unfortunately, mental disabilities were not treated to any great extent and remained stigmatized, a sad state of affairs which is still true to a great extent even today.

World War II and the Korean war again saw great loss of life but an increased rate of survival as medical practices improved. The Vietnam war and its long-lasting reverberations saw an increased awareness of the mental stress of war, and psychological disabilities became common knowledge. Unfortunately, these were not well-treated. However, the terms 'flashback' and 'post-traumatic stress disorder', and what they implied, became common knowledge. A variety of television shows and movies shed a bright light on how soldiers and civilians suffer during a war and that these effects did not end at the conclusion of it.

As important as the medical advances were for survival of the injured, this focus on a medical or disease model has created problems for us in the field of rehabilitation. Physiological problems were not handled well because the advances had been in surgical techniques and disease management. Essentially, surgeons had learned how to better amputate limbs, cut out foreign objects, administer antibiotics, sew up wounds, etc., without introducing an infection to the patient. There had been no, or very limited, advances in dealing with the emotional after-effects of sustaining and surviving such trauma. This problem exists to this day. The overdependence on the medical model with its focus on finding and removing pathology is insufficient for effective rehabilitation. While excellent medical treatment is necessary for survival, medical specialists should be eased out of the treatment picture once their skills are no longer appropriate. Instead, we continue to rely on medical opinion late into the rehabilitation process long after it is no longer relevant.

Take, for example, the case of Tom. Tom is a 28-year-old sheet-metal worker. He was very proud of his ability to do very accurate and demanding work. He sustained a serious crush injury to his leg when he was caught between a forklift lorry and its load. He was very angry at his co-worker. There had been a great deal of confusion at the worksite, first aid was delayed and he suffered a great deal of pain before help arrived. He had compound fractures, lacerations, etc. Medical treatment was routine except that the cast was placed too tightly and he developed gangrene. This was caught and treated but his leg never recovered and now has severe muscle wasting. He can bear his own weight for short periods of time but his career in sheet-metal work or any physical labour is over. The medical opinion was that he was lucky to be alive and that he should get back to work. And that's it. Tom tried, workers' compensation paid for some training, and he was sent to a work-conditioning programme but he did not progress.

Eventually Tom was referred to a psychologist who was able to determine the following. Tom was a physical kind of guy. He had liked to work out and had been proud of his body. He had been an excellent baseball player with hopes of going professional. He had a beautiful girlfriend and they had been planning on getting married. They had delayed the wedding and he was concerned that his relationship was in trouble because of his physical deformity. He was now extremely depressed and thinking that at the age of 28 his life was over. The psychologist was able to develop a comprehensive treatment plan in conjunction with the rehabilitation clinic he was attending. Along with physiotherapy, the psychologist was able to address Tom's issues with body image, self-esteem and the fears over his relationship, as well as loss issues related to the decrease of his physical prowess. Everything was going well, Tom's mood was improving and he was looking at career alternatives. He was on the road to recovery. Then the Workers' Compensation Board decided to speed things up and called him in for a medical assessment. There a physician of some type (there is no requirement in most Workers' Compensation Boards that they be physical medicine specialists) assessed him and concluded that he had reached a medical plateau and could return to work of some type. The Board then, in rapid succession, decided that he had had enough treatment, that his wage rate was such that he could access some type of employment and rapidly moved to terminate his benefits. This decision was made based on the opinion of a physician who had not been involved in the case and who saw Tom for at most an hour. Tom did not go back to work. His condition rapidly deteriorated and he sought legal representation. One year later he was still fighting with the Workers' Compensation Board, he was an emotional wreck, he had split up with his girlfriend and he was diagnosed with clinical depression. This case illustrates what can happen when we continue to make decisions based on medical opinion when medical opinion is no longer relevant. We do not ask a plumber to fix an electrical problem, yet we continue to ask physicians to provide opinions on issues outside their areas of expertise.

In this case this physician ignored all other evidence accumulated by the treatment team and rendered an individual opinion, and then the system acted on this opinion. How is this possible? The system places ultimate authority with this physician because we as a society are still fully subscribed to the medical model. Unfortunately the medical model, and physicians trained in this model, is not designed to deal with ongoing emotional issues and it is these issues that most often influence successful rehabilitation outcomes.

There have been attempts at more enlightened medical model approaches. For example, several workers' compensation providers have experimented with what may be generically referred to as a 'continuum of care'. The theory is that injured workers enter the continuum early in their recovery and progress through it with resources being added until such time as they can return to work or the system deems that it is done with them. The workers would enter the continuum as soon as it was known that they would not return to work within a short length of time. This period varied within jurisdictions but was placed in such a way to allow for spontaneous recovery to occur in order to avoid bringing these into the continuum. All stages were a maximum of six weeks long. Upon failure or lack of progress the person was moved to the next stage which escalated and intensified the treatment. The first stage of the continuum was often referred to as 'work conditioning' and essentially amounted to an exercise therapy programme. This stage was usually staffed by kinesiologists who supervised the exercise and tried to tailor the activities to the work that the person was going to be returning to. The desired outcome during this stage was a return to work (RTW), usually graduated, before the end of the six weeks. If the workers were unsuccessful they were moved to a more intensive treatment programme under the supervision of a physiotherapist. Again, primarily exercise-based, some education was now also provided. If there was still no success another stage was available which now included the services of a psychologist. If this stage failed, workers could be referred to a chronic pain treatment programme or, if it was determined that there were still some unresolved medical problems, to a medical rehabilitation programme under the supervision of a physician. If they were still not able to return to work they were sent for a pension assessment or deemed fit to return to some type of employment (Fig. 11.1).

This model has a great deal of potential but falls short in one critical area. The focus was on medical treatment until Stage 3 and by this time non-RTW behaviours and attitudes are well entrenched. This is essentially a failure-driven model. If medical treatment fails, treatment is intensified until it is

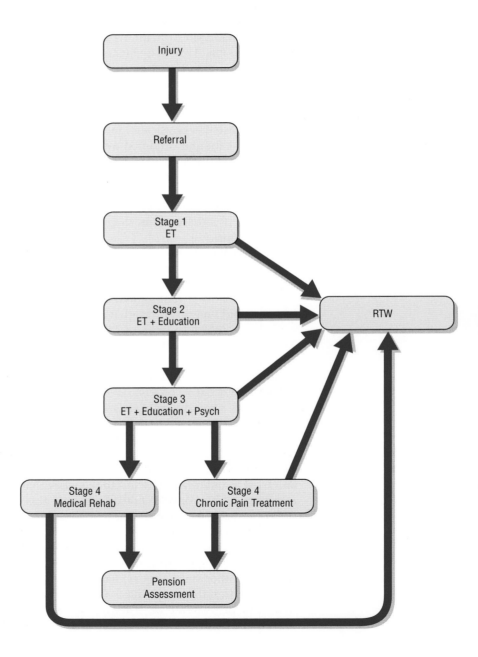

Figure 11.1 Stage model: continuum of care.

ing work in the person's life and which recognize that survival is not enough. Treatment needs to focus on the maintenance of self-esteem, the impact on the extended system and the maintenance of a worker construct, in other words all of the psychosocial factors that it is agreed are important but rarely receive treatment attention. This new approach will require that the medical model be limited to dealing with the person during their physical recovery period. It is our proposal that the overall treatment paradigm be referred to as comprehensive disability management and that the medical model be only one part of the process. Figure 11.2 illustrates this approach.

Figure 11.2 Comprehensive disability management.

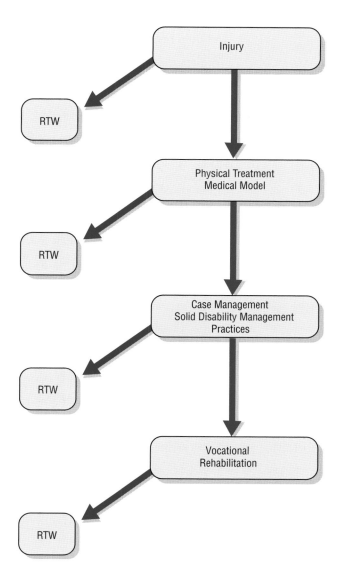

CONCLUSION

It is clear from World Health Organization data (2004) that psychological disabilities and psychological sequelae are growing at an alarming pace. It is imperative that we leave the narrow focus of medical treatment paradigms behind in order to develop new treatment paradigms based on an epistemological development of comprehensive treatment protocols that embrace non-medical solutions to non-medical problems. A narrow focus on physiological treatment has not served us well in the past (or in the present) and will not do so in the future. There is a saying that when one is carrying a hammer everything looks like a nail. The hammer is traditional rehabilitation but there are no nails. Individuals with disabilities, regardless of their aetiologies, require appropriate treatments not just medical rehabilitation because that is all we have. New treatments must be developed and funded so that people with disabilities can get the appropriate treatments and then benefit from this to become or stay fully participating members of society.

REFERENCES

Anderson T 1975 An alternative frame of reference for rehabilitation: the helping process versus the medical model. Archives of Physical Medicine and Rehabilitation 56:101–104

Cottone R, Emener W G 1990 The psychomedical paradigm of vocational rehabilitation and its alternatives. Rehabilitation Counseling Bulletin 34(2):91–103

Harder H G, Potts L 2002 Disability management: the insurance company of British Columbia experience. In: Murer E, Niederer P, Rumo-Jungo A et al (eds) Whiplash Associated Disorders: Medical, biomechanical and legal aspects. Staempfli, Bern, pp 133–150

Maki D R 1986 Foundations of applied rehabilitation counseling. In: Riggar T F, Maki D R, Wolf A W (eds) Applied Rehabilitation Counseling. Springer, New York

Stubbins J 1982 The clinical attitude in rehabilitation: a cross-cultural view. World Rehabilitation Fund, New York

World Health Organization 2004 The World Health Report 2004 – Changing history. WHO, Geneva http://www.who.int/whr/en/

Wright G N 1980 Total Rehabilitation. Little, Brown, New York

Chapter **12**

Duty to accommodate

LEARNING OBJECTIVES

- Acquire knowledge regarding the duty to accommodate in the disability management process
- Understand the legislative underpinnings of the duty to accommodate
- Understand the jurisprudence regarding the duty to accommodate
- Understand the employers', unions' and workers' responsibilities under the duty to accommodate
- Gain an accurate understanding of the costs of accommodation
- Gain some specific strategies for arranging accommodations in the workplace

INTRODUCTION

The duty to accommodate is based on legislation that has developed over the latter part of the last century. In 1948, the United Nations developed international agreements (UN 1948) which stated that:

- Everyone has a right to work, to free choice of employment, to just and favourable conditions of work and to protection against unemployment.
- Everyone, without discrimination, has the right to equal pay for equal work.

The United Nations followed this in 1975 with the 'Declaration of the Rights of Disabled Persons' (UN 1975) which stated, in part, that:

- Disabled people are entitled to the measures designed to enable them to become as self-reliant as possible.
- Disabled people have the right to medical, psychological and functional treatment, including prosthetic and orthotic appliances, to medical and social rehabilitation, aid, counselling, placement services and other services which will enable them to develop their capabilities and skills to the maximum and will hasten the process of their social integration or re-integration.
- Disabled people have the right to economic and social security and to a decent level of living. They have the right, according to their capabilities,

to secure and retain employment or to engage in a useful, productive and remunerative occupation, and to join trade unions.

- Disabled people are entitled to have their special needs taken into consideration at all stages of economic and social planning.
- Disabled people shall be protected against all exploitation, all regulations and all treatment of a discriminatory, abusive or degrading nature.

LEGISLATION

In Canada, the Canadian Charter of Rights, the Canadian Human Rights Act and the Employment Equity Act clearly identify the responsibility for accommodation. The Canadian Charter of Rights and Freedoms (CCRF) states:

> *Every individual is equal before and under the law and has the right to the equal protection and equal benefit of the law without discrimination and, in particular, without discrimination based on race, national or ethnic origin, colour, religion, sex, age or mental or physical disability.*
>
> (CCRF 1982: Section 15)

The Canadian Human Rights Act states:

> *The purpose of this Act is to extend the laws in Canada to give effect, within the purview of matters coming within the legislative authority of Parliament, to the principle that all individuals should have an opportunity equal with other individuals to make for themselves the lives that they are able and wish to have and to have their needs accommodated, consistent with their duties and obligations as members of society, without being hindered in or prevented from doing so by discriminatory practices based on race, national or ethnic origin, colour, religion, age, sex, sexual orientation, marital status, family status, disability or conviction for an offence for which a pardon has been granted.*
>
> (Canadian Human Rights Act 1985: Section 2)

The Employment Equity Act speaks on this issue in two sections. Section 5 states:

> *Every employer shall implement employment equity by*
>
> a. *identifying and eliminating employment barriers against people in designated groups that result from the employer's employment systems, policies and practices that are not authorized by law; and*
>
> b. *instituting such positive policies and practices and making such reasonable accommodations as will ensure that people in designated groups achieve a degree of representation in each occupational group in the employer's workforce that reflects their representation in*
>
>   i.   *the Canadian workforce, or*
>
>   ii. *those segments of the Canadian workforce that are identifiable by qualification, eligibility or geography and from which the employer may reasonably be expected to draw employ.*

Section 10 states that:

The employer shall prepare an employment equity plan that

a. *specifies the positive policies and practices that are to be instituted by the employer in the short term for the hiring, training, promotion and retention of people in designated groups and for the making of reasonable accommodations for those people, to correct the underrepresentation of those people identified by the analysis under paragraph 9(1)(a);*

b. *specifies the measures to be taken by the employer in the short term for the elimination of any employment barriers identified by the review under paragraph 9(1)(b);*

c. *establishes a timetable for the implementation of the matters referred to in paragraphs* (a) *and* (b);

d. *where underrepresentation has been identified by the analysis, establishes short term numerical goals for the hiring and promotion of people in designated groups in order to increase their representation in each occupational group in the workforce in which underrepresentation has been identified and sets out measures to be taken in each year to meet those goals;*

e. *sets out the employer's longer term goals for increasing the representation of people in designated groups in the employer's workforce and the employer's strategy for achieving those goals; and*

f. *provides for any other matter that may be prescribed.*

Each province within Canada also has provincial human rights statutes which deal with the duty to accommodate to some degree.

Three cases in Canadian jurisprudence speak on this issue. In order to understand the implications of these cases we must first understand how a Bona Fide Occupational Requirement or a Bona Fide Justification (BFJ) is established. These terms have historically only been applied to cases of direct discrimination. Direct discrimination is defined as:

Standards or policies that are discriminatory on their face, i.e., that clearly make an adverse distinction on the basis of a prohibited ground. For example, a policy that restricts a particular job to men could be characterised as prima facie direct discrimination as it specifically denies women an employment opportunity. Similarly, an employment standard requiring 20:20 uncorrected vision could be characterised as direct discrimination on the basis of disability as it specifically excludes people with vision impairments.

(Canadian Human Rights Commission 2003)

If it is established that an employer's policy or standard is direct discrimination then the employer must prove that this policy or standard is a bona-fide occupational requirement (Canadian Human Rights Commission 2003). In order to prove this the employer has to show that the standard or policy was:

■ imposed honestly and in good faith and was not imposed to undermine human rights legislation (the subjective element)

- reasonably necessary for the safe and efficient performance of the work and was not an unreasonable burden on those to whom it applied (the objective element).

Indirect or adverse effect discrimination is defined as:

> *standards or policies that are neutral on their face, i.e., that are applied equally to all people without distinction on a prohibited ground, but which nonetheless have an adverse effect based on a prohibited ground. For example, a job description which requires applicants to have a driver's license is neutral on its face as it does not specifically exclude anyone. It is not neutral in its effect, however: people who cannot get a driver's license because of vision impairments or epilepsy, for example, would be precluded from applying for the job.*
>
> (Canadian Human Rights Commission 2003)

Again, if it is established that an employer's policy or standard had an adverse effect on a group then the employer would have to prove two points (Canadian Human Rights Commission 2003):

- that there was a rational connection between the job and the standard or policy
- that it was not possible to accommodate the specific complainant without incurring undue hardship.

In 1998 the Canadian Parliament narrowed the gap between these two definitions when it passed amendments to the Canadian Human Rights Act (1985). By doing this Parliament made it clear that employers had a duty to accommodate individuals who were discriminated against by any policy or practice. Section 15 of the Canadian Human Rights Act now reads:

> *For any practice mentioned in paragraph (1)(a) to be considered to be based on a bona fide occupational requirement and for any practice mentioned in paragraph (1)(g) to be considered to have a bona fide justification, it must be established that accommodation of the needs of an individual or a class of individuals affected would impose undue hardship on the person who would have to accommodate those needs, considering health, safety and cost.*

For completeness and clarification section (1)(*a*) states:

> *It is not a discriminatory practice if any refusal, exclusion, expulsion, suspension, limitation, specification or preference in relation to any employment is established by an employer to be based on a* bona fide *occupational requirement*

and (1)(*g*) states:

> *It is not a discriminatory practice in the circumstances described in section 5 or 6, an individual is denied any goods, services, facilities or accommodation or access thereto or occupancy of any commercial premises or residential accommodation or is a victim of any adverse differentiation and there is* bona fide *justification for that denial or differentiation.*

What is meant by 'undue hardship'?

The Ontario Human Rights Commission (2004), in a fact sheet, states that only three factors can be considered when defining undue hardship. These are:

- cost
- outside sources of funding
- health and safety.

The Commission goes on to say that a cost is 'undue' if it is so high that it changes the essential nature of the business or if it affects the survival of the organization or business as a whole. The business must be able to quantify these costs. There is room for some flexibility depending on the size of the employer. What may be an 'undue cost' for a small employer may not be undue hardship for a larger one. If the accommodation requires the business to fundamentally change the nature of what it does, this may also constitute undue hardship.

An employer must also consider and attempt to access outside sources of funding. This may include federal and provincial government programmes which may offset some of the costs of the accommodation. If the cost is too large to undertake all at once, the employer should consider phasing it in over time.

An employer may argue that health and safety factors may limit the accommodation that is possible. Before this can be argued, it must first be decided whether any applicable health and safety requirements can be waived or modified, or if alternatives can be found to protect the health and safety of the workforce. As long as no one else is put at risk, it is acceptable for people with disabilities to take on some degree of risk, provided they are fully informed of that risk.

Case study   Bhinder vs. Canadian National Railway Company

In 1985 the Supreme Court of Canada decided Bhinder vs. Canadian National Railway Company (CN) (SCR 1985). CN introduced a work rule that all employees must wear a hard hat at a particular worksite. Bhinder, a Sikh employee, refused to comply because his religion prohibited wearing headgear other than the turban. Consequently Bhinder was dismissed since the company refused to make exceptions to the rule and Bhinder refused to accept other work not requiring a hard hat. The Canadian Human Rights Tribunal found that CN had engaged in a discriminatory practice and ordered reinstatement and compensation for loss of salary. The Federal Court of Appeal set aside that decision and referred the matter back for disposition on the basis that the work rule was not a discriminatory practice. At issue here was whether or not the hard hat rule was a bona-fide occupational requirement.

Case study   The Meiorin case

In 1999 the Supreme Court of Canada decided what has become known as the Meiorin case which is appropriately referred to as the British Columbia Government and Service Employees' Union vs. The Government of the Province of British Columbia as represented by the Public Service Employee Relations Commission (SCR 1999a). This case has become the benchmark when considering the duty to accommodate. The facts of the case are as follows:

1. Ms Meiorin was employed for three years by the British Columbia Ministry of Forests as part of an Initial Attack Forest Firefighting Crew. Ms Meiorin's supervisors found her work to be satisfactory.
2. Ms Meiorin was not asked to take a physical fitness test until 1994, when she was required to pass the Government's 'Bona Fide Occupational Fitness Tests and Standards for BC Forest Service Wildland Firefighters'.
3. The tests were developed in response to a Coroner's inquest report that recommended that only physically fit employees be assigned as frontline forest firefighters for safety reasons.
4. Two methodological issues are critical to this case. First, the research was primarily descriptive, based on measuring the average performance levels of the test subjects and converting these data into minimum performance standards. Second, it did not seem to distinguish between the male and female test subjects.
5. Ms Meiorin tried four times to pass the test but failed to meet the aerobic standard. As a result her employment was terminated.
6. Evidence accepted by the arbitrator demonstrated that, owing to physiological differences, most women have a lower aerobic capacity than most men. Even with training, most women cannot increase their aerobic capacity to the level required by the aerobic standard, although training can allow most men to meet it.
7. There was no credible evidence showing that the prescribed aerobic capacity was necessary for either men or women to perform the work of a forest firefighter satisfactorily. On the contrary, Ms Meiorin had in the past performed her work well, without apparent risk to herself, her colleagues or the public.

The arbitrator concluded that Ms Meiorin had established a prima-facie case of adverse effect discrimination by showing that the aerobic standard has a disproportionately negative effect on women. He also found that the Government had presented no credible evidence that Ms Meiorin's inability to meet the aerobic standard meant that she constituted a safety risk to herself, her colleagues or the public, and hence had not discharged its burden of showing that it had accommodated Ms Meiorin to the point of undue hardship. He ordered that she be reinstated to her former position and compensated for her lost wages and benefits.

The Government appealed against this decision. On appeal the arbitrator's decision was overruled on the basis that so long as the standard is necessary to the safe and efficient performance of the work and is applied through individualized testing, there is no discrimination. The Court of Appeal read the arbitrator's reasons as finding that the aerobic standard was necessary for the safe and efficient performance of the work. This was in fact an error as the arbitrator had made no such conclusion and so the Supreme Court of Canada upheld the arbitrator's initial decision.

The Supreme Court also made some suggestions as to what employers should ask themselves before responding to an employee's request for an accommodation (SCR 1999a: Section 65). These were:

■ Has the employer investigated alternative approaches that do not have a discriminatory effect, such as individual testing against a more individually sensitive standard?
■ If alternative standards were investigated and found to be capable of fulfilling the employer's purpose, why were they not implemented?
■ Is it necessary to have *all* employees meet the single standard for the employer to accomplish its legitimate purpose or could standards reflective of group or individual differences and capabilities be established?

■ Is there a way to do the job that is less discriminatory while still accomplishing the employer's legitimate purpose?

■ Is the standard properly designed to ensure that the desired qualification is met without placing an undue burden on those to whom the standard applies?

■ Have other parties who are obliged to assist in the search for possible accommodation fulfilled their roles? The task of determining how to accommodate individual differences may also place burdens on the employee and, if there is a collective agreement, a union.

Employers were also required to engage in a four-step process to ensure that their efforts were serious and conscientious:

1. Determine if employees are capable of performing tasks in their own occupations.
2. If not, determine if employees can perform the tasks in their own occupations if these tasks are modified or reorganized.
3. If not, determine if employees can perform different jobs outside their occupations.
4. If not, determine if employees can perform different jobs outside their occupations in a modified or reorganized form.

The employer has an obligation to engage in this process up to the point of undue hardship.

Case study   The Grismer case

Just three months after the Meiorin decision the Supreme Court issued its decision in British Columbia (Superintendent of Motor Vehicles) vs. British Columbia (Council of Human Rights) or the Grismer case. Mr Grismer had homonymous hemianopia (HH) which eliminated most of his left-side peripheral vision in both eyes. The BC Superintendent of Motor Vehicles cancelled his driver's licence on the grounds that his vision no longer met the standard of a minimum field of vision of 120 degrees. Certain exceptions to this standard were allowed but people with HH were not permitted to hold a driver's licence in BC.

Mr Grismer reapplied several times and passed all tests except the field of vision test. He was not permitted to demonstrate that he could compensate for his lost vision. He filed a complaint with the BC Council of Human Rights and was successful on the basis that the Superintendent of Motor Vehicles had failed to prove that there was a BFJ for the standard applied to people with HH.

This decision was appealed against and, on appeal, the Supreme Court of Canada held that the findings in the Meiorin case were equally applicable in service provision cases. In doing so the court asked these questions:

■ Is the discriminatory practice or policy rationally connected to the function being performed?

■ Did the service provider adopt the particular standard with an honest and good-faith belief that it was necessary for the fulfilment of its purpose or goal?

■ Is the standard reasonably necessary for the service provider to accomplish its purpose or goal?

Given the importance of this finding to people with disabilities it is important to hear directly from Justice McLachlin who said (SCR 1999b: 868):

> This case is not about whether unsafe drivers must be allowed to drive. There is no suggestion that a visually impaired driver should be licensed unless she or he can compensate for the impairment and drive safely. Rather, this case is about whether, on the evidence before the Member, Mr Grismer should have been given a chance to prove through an individual assessment that he could drive. It is also about combating false assumptions regarding the effects of disabilities on individual capacities. All too often, people with disabilities are assumed to be unable to accomplish certain tasks based on the experience of able-bodied individuals. The thrust of human rights legislation is to eliminate such assumptions and break down the barriers that stand in the way of equality for all.

IMPLICATIONS

This legislation and jurisprudence provides the basis for the protection and integration of individuals with disabilities into the workforce and is used to ensure that employers make accommodations as required. What then are the implications for an employer given this new reality?

The issue of financial costs seems fairly straightforward. The employer is required to pay for an accommodation up to the point of undue hardship. However, this can be mitigated by additional factors. Most often the size of the organization is used as a determining factor but this is too simplistic an approach. Other factors must also be considered, for example the general economic climate of the society the employer is functioning in and the overall financial health of the organization must be considered, not only its size. For example, on the surface it may seem that the installation of a lift may be a minor matter to a large organization but it may bankrupt a smaller organization thereby qualifying as undue hardship. If the smaller employer, however, is very wealthy or if the larger employer near bankruptcy, this may change the finding on which organization may be able to invoke undue hardship. Also, if external funds are available, through a WCB for example, these funds should be accessed to facilitate the accommodation.

In some instances employee morale may be used as rationale for declaring undue hardship. However, the Supreme Court of Canada has ruled that only employee objections based on well-grounded concerns about the violation of rights should be considered. Cases involving employee morale that have been supported in the courts are those where employees are required to work constant overtime because of the continued absence of an employee with a disability.

Another important consideration is with regard to the health and safety of other employees. The courts and arbitrators have given the safety of others more weight than the safety of the injured employee. However, substantial evidence is required to prove that accommodation will adversely affect the safety of other employees. Risk to the employee and others should be assessed considering four factors (Dyck 2000):

- the nature of the risk
- the severity of the risk
- the probability of the risk
- the scope of the risk.

It should be noted that the employee and the union also have a duty to accommodate. This was clearly outlined in the case of Central Okanagan School District No. 23 vs. Renaud. Renaud was a Seventh Day Adventist whose Sabbath is from dusk on Friday to dusk on Saturday. The normal working shift was Monday to Friday. The employer suggested a Sunday to Thursday shift for him. However, this was in contravention of the collective agreement and the union refused to make an exception. Renaud refused to report to work on a Friday afternoon and was fired. He appealed and won. The union was obliged to accommodate the schedule offered by the employer. In summary the Justices stated (SCR 1992: 970):

Here, the union had a shared duty, arising out of the adverse effect dis-crimination, to accommodate the appellant. The employer did not need to explore all other reasonable accommodations. The proposal presented to the union was reasonable. The union, therefore, was jointly liable with the employer. The search for accommodation is a multi-party inquiry. The complainant also has a duty to assist in securing an appropriate accom-modation and his or her conduct must therefore be considered in deter-mining whether the duty to accommodate has been fulfilled. When an employer has initiated a proposal that is reasonable and would, if imple-mented, fulfill the duty to accommodate, the complainant has a duty to facilitate the implementation of the proposal. If the complainant fails to take reasonable steps and causes the proposal to founder, the complaint will be dismissed. The complainant is also obligated to accept reasonable accom-modation and the employer's duty is discharged if a proposal that would be reasonable in all the circumstances is turned down. The complainant did all that could be expected of him in this case.

When considering accommodation in the workplace, it should be noted that an employer is not required to create new positions within the organi-zation in order to accommodate an employee. This also means that having the employee doing some of the duties of their original job and adding some other duties is not the preferred approach. The person should be placed in a job in which they can perform all the essential demands, with accommo-dation as required. The work must be productive and meaningful work that supports the organization's objectives. There is also no obligation to displace another employee from an occupied job in order to accommodate an injured worker.

How, then, does an employer or a union ensure that it is upholding the duty-to-accommodate legislation? Suggestions include:

- keeping up to date with evolving legislation, policies and jurisprudence
- knowing the jobs at your worksite and what the job requirements are
- arranging for an appropriate assessment of the individual's short-term and long-term abilities post-injury or -illness
- knowing the different types of accommodation that are available
- developing a policy on accommodation
- developing a team approach to problem-solving
- being flexible.

APPLICATION

The next section of this chapter will examine methods of accommodation for both physical and mental impairments and provide examples of accommodation.

Job accommodation can be defined as any modification in a workplace or workplace procedure that enables a person to do their job. Generally, accom-modations are made for an employee with a disability. However, a 2001 Statistics Canada survey found that only 4% of disabled employees required physical changes to the workplace.

More than half of all accommodations cost less than Can$500. Examples of inexpensive modifications include (HRDC 2002):

■ provision of a telephone headset
■ ergonomic chairs
■ replacement of a computer mouse with a trackball system.

Examples of more extensive accommodations usually involve making a worksite accessible for people with mobility disabilities. These may involve (HRDC 2002):

■ accessible corridors
■ ramps with proper grading and handrails
■ wider doorways
■ provision of adequate parking spaces.

More frequently than ever before worksites are coming to grips with the need to accommodate people with mental health problems. The needs of these people may require different accommodations than those with physical difficulties, and more creativity and flexibility may be required. Mental health issues are frequently very sensitive and great care must be taken not to worsen the situation by inadvertent disclosure of information or the reinforcing of stereotypical images.

Examples of accommodations for people with mental health issues include (HRDC 2002):

■ flexible scheduling
■ job-sharing
■ more frequent breaks
■ the provision of private work spaces to reduce distractions
■ use of calendars or electronic organizers
■ documenting expectations in writing.

Vision impairments, especially as the population ages, are becoming more common in the workplace. Accommodation of those with visual impairments requires flexibility as the level of visual acuity can vary greatly. There are accommodations available such as handheld magnifiers, large-screen computer monitors, Braille devices, audible devices and guide dogs (HRDC 2002). Most countries have groups that assist people with visual impairments and advocate for their needs. Groups such as the Canadian Institute for the Blind can be excellent resources for determining the kind of accommodation required.

Another impairment becoming more frequent in worksites as the population ages is hearing impairment. This condition varies from total deafness to a great variety of lesser degrees of hearing loss. Individuals who have or sustain hearing loss will require accommodation. However, the type of accommodation will depend on the type of hearing loss and whether it is going to deteriorate further or is at its most severe. Useful assistive technologies include hearing aids, the removal of extraneous noise from the work environment, email or other written communication, assistive listening devices such as TTY phones (text telephones), and sign-language interpreters. It is critical to ensure that the person is not placed at risk by not being able to hear safety warnings. Consequently, special attention should be paid to warning and emergency systems in the workplace.

Providing assistance to people with substance addictions is fairly well-defined within most Canadian workplaces. It should be noted that these addictions have been defined as disabilities and consequently require accommodation. Simply referring someone to an employee assistance programme is not sufficient. An employer must also consider accommodations such as providing time off for treatment, or modifications to work hours to allow the person to attend counselling or support groups, for example.

As disability management (DM) branches out to work with all people with disabilities (not just those acquired at work) it will be necessary to become familiar with all types of disabilities including learning and developmental disabilities.

People with learning disabilities can have a wide range of needs and require individual specific accommodation. For example, one person with dyslexia who has learned to compensate may need nothing except a little more time to read instructions, while another person whose dyslexia is more severe may not be able to compensate and will need more extensive accommodation.

Examples of developmental disabilities include Down's syndrome, cerebral palsy and autism. People with these conditions can vary substantially in their ability to function. However, certain difficulties – such as difficulty with reading, writing, mathematics and problem-solving – are common. For these individuals, a successful accommodation has been to provide job coaches who help them learn the essential job tasks, adjust to work routines, and establish relationships with supervisors and co-workers. Depending on the severity of the disability some of these individuals may eventually function without a job coach while others may need to have access to a coach on a regular and permanent basis.

Traumatic brain injuries cross this divide between physical and mental issues since the consequences of the brain injury can include both mental and physical impairment.

People with such disabilities often require both the more traditional 'physical' accommodation as well as a non-traditional, perhaps mental-health-related, accommodation. For example, acquired traumatic brain injuries typically affect the frontal and temporal lobes of the brain, which can result in changes in thought processes, behaviour and personality. Observable changes may include physical limitations, behavioural changes, impulse control problems, and visual and memory problems. Accommodations may include reducing distractions and interruptions, breaking tasks into smaller assignments, and using cueing strategies such as calendars and notebooks. Reassignment to a position that involves less contact with others may also be required.

The types of accommodation used in industry will vary widely and often require creative solutions that draw on the expertise of the injured/ill employee, co-workers and supervisors, and healthcare providers.

CONCLUSION

This chapter has outlined the legislation, jurisprudence and policies in Canada that support the duty to accommodate employees with disabilities in the workplace and has provided definitions for the terms 'undue hardship' and 'bona-fide occupational requirements'. We have provided examples of the types of impairments that may require accommodation and some brief strategies for how to proceed. It is our hope that this discussion, though based on the Canadian experience, will provide a basis for discussing accommodation issues throughout the world, thereby assisting employers, unions and DM professionals in developing solutions for meeting the needs of people with disabilities.

REFERENCES

Canadian Charter of Rights and Freedoms 1982 http://laws.justice.gc.ca/en/charter/
Canadian Human Rights Act 1985 http://laws.justice.gc.ca/en/H-6/
Canadian Human Rights Commission 2003
    http://www.chrc-ccdp.ca/discrimination/occupational-en.asp#top
Dyck D 2000 Disability Management: Theory, strategy and industry practice. Butterworth, Markham, Ontario
Employment Equity Act 1995 http://laws.justice.gc.ca/en/E-5.401/
Human Resources and Development Canada 2002 Advancing the Inclusion of Persons with Disabilities http://www.hrsdc.gc.ca/asp/gateway.asp?hr=en/hip/odi/documents/advancingInclusion/aipdIndex.shtml&hs=pyp (later Human Resources and Skills Development Canada)
Ontario Human Rights Commission 2004
    http://www.ohrc.on.ca/english/publications/disability-policy-fact4.shtml
Statistics Canada 2001 Participation and Activity Limitation Survey
    http://stcwww.statcan.ca/english/sdds/3251.htm
Supreme Court of Canada 1985
    http://www.lexum.umontreal.ca/csc-scc/en/pub/1985/vol2/html/1985scr2_0561.html
Supreme Court of Canada 1992 http://www.lexum.umontreal.ca/csc-scc/en/pub/1992/vol2/html/1992scr2_0970.html
Supreme Court of Canada 1999a Meiorin Case http://www.lexum.umontreal.ca/csc-scc/en/pub/1999/vol3/html/1999scr3_0003.html
Supreme Court of Canada 1999b Grismer Case http://www.lexum.umontreal.ca/csc-scc/en/pub/1999/vol3/html/1999scr3_0868.htm
United Nations 1948 The Universal Declaration of Human Rights. Office of the High Commission on Human Rights http://www.unhchr.ch/udhr/
United Nations 1975 Declaration on the Rights of Disabled Persons
    http://www.unhchr.ch/html/menu3/b/72.htm

Chapter **13**

Programme evaluation

LEARNING OBJECTIVES

- Understand the evaluation process
- Know how to establish an evaluation programme
- Be able to perform a cost–benefit analysis
- Recognize the importance of quantifying return on investment

INTRODUCTION

A great deal of goodwill surrounded the start of the first disability management (DM) programmes. Employers, unions and others joined together to do what was perceived to be the 'right thing'. In much of the initial public relations material, DM was touted as a 'win win win' situation referring to the process allowing the worker, the employer and the unions to all be winners. As noble as this may have been, goodwill is never enough to sustain a business or a programme. Sooner or later there is going to have to be proof that the programme delivers what was promised. It should be noted that DM programmes are not being singled out by this requirement. It is part of an organization's responsibility to show that it is responsible in all that it does, including the provision of DM services. In fact, many organizations have been convinced by the promise of financial savings to introduce DM programmes. How then should a DM programme be evaluated?

METHODOLOGY

Given the desire to do the 'right thing' and the urgency to do it, organizations do not always plan how to evaluate a programme before it begins. Some people, in fact, believe evaluation is a useless activity that generates lots of boring data with useless conclusions. All too frequently this has been true in the past. It was not uncommon to choose programme evaluation methods largely on the basis of achieving complete scientific accuracy, reliability and validity. This approach often generated extensive research data from which very carefully chosen conclusions were drawn; generalizations and recommendations were avoided. As a result, evaluation reports tended to reiterate the obvious and left programme administrators disappointed and sceptical about the value of evaluation in general. Fortunately, this is changing and programme evaluation is focusing more on utility, relevance and practicality while still maintaining scientific credibility.

Programme evaluation is not about proving the success or failure of a programme. This premise would assume that the programme is planned and implemented perfectly the first time it is offered and never needs any feedback in order to improve. Programme evaluation is established to provide an ongoing means of continuous improvement. Programmes need quantitative data results and qualitative responses from participants and stakeholders to improve over time. Proper programme evaluation provides this information.

It is a commonly held belief that evaluation is a highly unique and complex process that occurs at a certain time in a certain way, and almost always includes the use of external experts. Many people believe they must be completely knowledgeable of all the statistical techniques and research methodologies to perform programme evaluation. But this is not so. In fact, as discussed in Van Beek and Kuvaja (2000), there is a growing expectation that services will be proven to be cost-effective and that organizations expect an attitude of continuous improvement. What they have to know is what they really need to know in order to decide if the programme is working. In other words, what constitutes success for the programme? This means taking the time to really understand what is happening and why. Programme evaluation is not just about the numbers but also about the process. Most organizations already collect most of the information to provide this kind of analysis but it is usually not in a form that is readily accessible or understandable.

There are three general types of programme evaluation: needs evaluation; formative evaluation; and summative evaluation.

Needs evaluation

The needs evaluation is carried out prior to the formation of the programme in order to identify what the current state of affairs are and what the actual needs are. Then the programme is designed to meet these needs and the measurable objectives outlined in the planning process. Such an evaluation should, of course, come first. However, many organizations, including those wishing to implement DM programmes, are in a hurry and all too frequently circumvent this process. The logic goes something like this: we know the needs, we know (anecdotally) that the programme works, so let's save some time and money and just do it. Unfortunately, such an approach may miss some critical needs, is vulnerable to being based only on what senior management thinks the needs are, and avoids the process of establishing a baseline against which further gains or losses can be measured.

In planning a DM programme, a needs evaluation seeks to answer questions such as:

- What is the profile of the group we are trying to serve?
- What is the current picture? Claim cost, rates, types, duration, etc.?
- What are the needs of the group with respect to DM?
- What will make a DM programme effective to the group?
- How will we know if the DM programme is being effective? What measures will we use?

Formative evaluation

A formative evaluation is completed after the programme has been running for some time in order to determine if it is functioning as intended and if it is meeting the needs of the group. A simple way of thinking about this is to ask if the programme is doing what the group thought it was going to do. If not, this evaluation makes recommendation on how the programme can be altered in order to meet the intended needs.

A formative evaluation of a DM programme asks the following types of question:

- Are enough people being referred to the programme?
- Are people aware of the programme?
- Are the referrals of the kind that were anticipated?
- Are the timelines for referral, treatment and return to work (RTW) being met?
- What are the bottlenecks in the system?
- Are the targets specific to communication being met (i.e. first contact)?
- Is the workload of the staff as planned?
- Are the staff working as they should?
- Do the staff have the resources, time and skills necessary to do the job?

Summative evaluation

A summative evaluation is conducted to determine the actual outcome of a programme. This is when evaluators measure changes against baseline data identified in the needs evaluation. If that did not happen then evaluators must determine, before beginning this evaluation, what the determinants of success are. These outcomes may vary by programme and by who is being asked. For example, the staff may have a very different view than the supervisors or the union. Consequently, it is critical to decide whose measure(s) of success will be used. Determining and agreeing upon the evaluation criteria beforehand can avoid a great deal of frustration at this stage.

A summative evaluation of a DM programme asks the following types of question:

- Are more people going back to work now than before the programme?
- Are people going back to work faster than before the programme?
- Are the insurance costs decreasing?
- Are grievances regarding the RTW process decreasing?
- Is this result caused by the programme?

Cost–efficiency

Often cost-effectiveness measures and cost-efficiency measures are part of this process. Cost-effectiveness simply asks the question: is the money that we are spending and the effort we are making buying us what we wanted? If the answer is 'Yes' then the next question is: can we do this in a more cost-efficient manner? This is a more specific matter and an assessment of cost-efficiency asks questions such as:

- Is the programme achieving its objectives at a reasonable cost?
- Can a comparison be made? That is, is this programme achieving the same or better level of success as another programme costing the same or less money?

Both of these criteria are complex to measure and will be covered later in this chapter.

There are other names for these evaluations. You may see references to terms such as 'goal-based assessment', 'process assessment', 'outcome assessment' and 'needs assessment'. All of these are covered in the above models of programme evaluation. The complexity and detail involved in any of the three evaluations mentioned above depend entirely on the type of questions being answered.

The order of these provides a logical sequence for conducting the evaluations. If need is not measured first, it is impossible to plan a programme appropriately. Without a properly planned, well-implemented programme there will be no meaningful outcomes. Without such outcomes there is no point in worrying if the programme is meeting its goals or if it is being delivered in a cost-effective manner (Wholey 1983).

GETTING STARTED

Frequently, there is a desire to know everything there is to know. However, with limited resources it is important to prioritize what is an absolute 'need to know' and what is a 'nice to know'. Then a decision can be made as to how to expend resources; if the 'need to know' is met then resources can be expended going after the 'nice to know'.

How the programme evaluation is planned depends on what information is needed in order to answer the questions asked. This is where the decision is made to go with a formative or summative evaluation (assuming it is too late for a needs evaluation). It is very important to be clear at this stage what each type of evaluation does. The expectations of the groups requesting the evaluation need to be identified and the type of evaluation selected accordingly. There are always compromises to be made. For example, someone will want more information and a broad range of factors and someone else will want less breadth and more detail. These disagreements need to be worked out to the satisfaction of all parties before the evaluation begins.

Here are some general questions that may help in setting up an evaluation:

- What is the purpose of the evaluation? That is, what questions have to be answered?
- Who is going to receive the information and what decisions will be based on the information?
- What kind of information is needed to make these decisions?
- From what sources should the information be collected? For example, employees, supervisors, medical treatment providers, users of the programme, etc.
- What is the best way to collect the information? For example, questionnaires, interviews, programme audit, observation and focus groups.
- What is the timeline for the evaluation?
- What resources (financial and human) are available to conduct the evaluation?

If it has been decided to complete a formative evaluation the following questions may be useful:

- On what basis is someone referred to the DM programme?
- What is required for the referral to take place?
- Is the referral occurring at the appropriate time?
- Are referral timelines, treatment and RTW achieved?
- Are the right kinds of people being referred?
- Are the staff adequately trained in order to fulfil their functions?
- Are the programme materials clear, easily understood and readily available?
- Does the programme have adequate resources?
- Is the programme adequately supported by both management and the union?
- Is everyone in the organization aware of the programme and what its goals are?
- What do the users, staff, employer, union, external stakeholders, etc. consider to be the strengths and weaknesses of the programme?
- What are the typical complaints heard from the users of the programme?
- What can be done to improve the programme?

Of course, these questions are examples only – the exact questions need to be designed uniquely for each programme.

If it has been determined that a summative evaluation should be conducted, the design and targeted outcomes must be clear. Summative evaluation may have the most dire consequences of any of the evaluations as a programme's resources may be terminated or decreased and people may lose their positions or even their jobs based on the outcomes. From a positive point of view, the summative evaluation may demonstrate the need for additional resources and investment in the programme. It is therefore imperative that such an evaluation be appropriately planned and implemented. The following form a series of steps that should be considered when setting up such an evaluation:

1. Identify the major outcomes that need to be evaluated. It is appropriate to ask what the mission of the programme is. If there is a mission statement, a review of that statement would be appropriate. For example, if the overall mission is to help people with disabilities RTW

post-injury or -illness then has this been happening? If this is not clear or if it appears that the mission has been confused or lost it would be appropriate to ask questions such as: what is the programme doing? Then list the activities and ask for each activity: why is it being done? The answer to this is usually some form of 'We are doing that because . . .', which in fact is an outcome and needs to be counted as such. For example, the mission statement of a DM programme may have said nothing about attendance management. However, upon examination it is revealed that a substantial amount of programme time is being allotted to this task. When asked why, the response may be 'We are doing attendance management because the Vice-President of human resources said that we have the skills to do it and no one else was doing it'. This may be true but if not identified as a mandate of the programme it will not be counted in the evaluation. This outcome may not be valued as it was not part of the original mission statement, and discarded in the future, or it may be valued and added to the mission of the programme. In any case it needs to be counted as an outcome of the programme.

2. Choose the most important outcomes and prioritize them. Make a decision as to how many answers your budgeted resources will buy.

3. For each outcome, specify the factors which will indicate that the desired outcomes are being reached. This is often the most important and enlightening step. However, it is often the most challenging step as a decision has to be made as to what really matters.

4. Specify who the participants are, i.e. everyone who has participated since the inception of the programme or only those in the first year, first three months or whatever period of time is desired. In larger programmes it may not be possible to evaluate every person's experience so a sample group must be created. For example, a multi-site programme may decide to do an evaluation based on a certain number of cases per site.

5. It is also a good idea to expand the evaluation to those people who were qualified to enter the programme but did not. Why didn't they enter the programme? Were they just as well off not going into the programme?

6. Determine what method or combination of methods will be used to gather the necessary information. Consider all types of methods such as a programme audit, documentation review, observation of the programme in operation, questionnaires, interviews, case studies, etc. An evaluation may be comprised of one or any combination of these methods.

7. Determine how the data will be analysed before you begin. A pilot study is always a good idea, just to make sure that the end result will be what was desired.

8. It helps to think about the structure of the final report before the evaluation begins. Thinking about what will need to be written up will help determine what goes into the evaluation.

The various types of data collection are listed in Table 13.1.

Table 13.1 Types of data collection

Methodology	Why it is used	Advantages	Disadvantages
Questionnaires or surveys	Anonymous response; less threatening to many people	• Can be completed anonymously • Easier to analyse statistically (software available) • May be able to use or adapt existing questionnaires	• Do not know who is filling it in • Cannot control the person's interpretation of the questions • May not achieve a large enough return to be meaningful
Interviews	When it is desired to fully understand someone's experiences of the programme	• Depth of information • Can probe and draw out more information	• Time-consuming • Labour-intensive • Potentially costly • Interviewer bias may be introduced
Documentation review	To gain an understanding of how a programme is keeping records and if the documentation matches what is stated	• Can achieve a clear understanding of the record-keeping of a programme • Does not interrupt participant's routine in the programme • Uses existing information – few biases about information	• Time-consuming • Information may be incomplete • Do not receive a complete picture • Dependent on existing data
Observation	Makes it possible to gather accurate information about how a programme actually operates, particularly human interactions, i.e. communication	• The evaluator is actually present during the operation of the programme • Allows direct, unfiltered observation	• Requires a trained observer who can interpret interactions • Time-consuming • Can be costly • Analysis is complex • Evaluator can influence behaviours of programme's participants simply by being present
Focus groups	• Makes it possible to explore a topic in depth through group discussion • Has the benefit of being able to explore preplanned questions as well as exploring issues raised by the participants	• Possible to acquire common impressions quickly • Possible to acquire information on specific, targeted issues	• Requires a trained facilitator • Requires specific-use facilities • Can be difficult to schedule
Case studies	Used to fully investigate the experiences of a few people in a programme	• Gathers in-depth information • Provides powerful information which can portray the actual experience of being in a programme	• Time-consuming • Requires a skilled researcher • Results cannot be generalized

ETHICS

Various organizations may require that an evaluation be vetted through their ethics review process. Even if this is not the case, it is a good idea to consider the ethical implications of completing an evaluation (see Chapter 15). At the very least if you are asking individuals for information you should make them completely aware of the reasons for the evaluation and ensure that they are willing participants. You may wish to have them sign an informed consent form. This form should be very clear and easy to understand so that the person can quickly gain an understanding of what you are asking them to do, what the bounds of confidentiality are, what is going to happen to the information collected and how the results will be shared.

COST-EFFECTIVENESS

Programme evaluation would not be complete without considering costs and cost savings. Recommendations for programme development, expansion or continuance, which are not accompanied by cost and saving estimates, will probably not be taken seriously in today's business environment. Additionally, being able to relate programme outcomes to costs is important to demonstrate the value of human services. Cost projections and programme objectives (potential savings) can assist in choosing the type and breadth of the programme.

There are many costs to quantify in running a programme. There are the costs that are borne simply to commence the programme. They include the cost of programme development such as policies, procedures and processes. These costs are spent no matter how many participants enter the programme.

Organizations will differ in which cost items they track. Some organizations do not include costs that they consider part of operating the business; others may include all costs. Some of the types of items that may be included are as follows.

Disability costs

- Sick leave cost
- Disability insurance premiums
- Workers' compensation premiums and adjustments.

Operating costs

- Salary and benefits
- Equipment – hardware and software
- Supplies
- Communication costs (telephone, email)
- Education information costs (developing information for supervisors, employees and service providers)
- Professional development (journals, updating)

- Infrastructure costs (cost involved in providing space, accounting, upper-level management and supervision, human resources assistance with recruitment, legal support, etc.).

Programme costs

- Third-party services – third-party administrator, Functional Ability Evaluations, Independent Medical Examinations, physiotherapy, other assessments
- Assistive devices and technologies
- Changes or renovations to the work environment or workstation
- Rehabilitation – on-the-job training (or other training)

Table 13.2 shows the budget for a DM department. We have not included costs such as maintenance, cleaning services or insurance costs as the company would pay these with or without this department area.

Table 13.2 Example of the budget for a disability management department

Department	Budget (US$)
Disability premiums	
Workers' compensation	4 000 000
Sick leave	5 000 000
Long-term disability	2 000 000
Employees' salaries	
Director	90 000
Managers	60 000
Coordinators	80 000
Administrator	30 000
Benefits (30% of salaries)	78 000
Co-op student	6000
Professional development	4000
Information sessions (training)	4000
Office	
Computer	7500
Software	1000
Filing cabinets	1000
Copying	4500
Telephone	12 000
Supplies	12 000
Infrastructure costs (space)	5000
External services	
Third-party administrator	300 000
Independent assessments	250 000
Rehabilitation services	100 000
Programme cost	**1 045 000**

Table 13.3 Simple cost–benefit analysis

	Premiums before programme (US$)	Premiums after programme (US$)	Savings (US$)
Workers' compensation	4 000 000	3 000 000	1 000 000
Sick leave	5 000 000	4 000 000	1 000 000
Long-term disability	2 000 000	1 800 000	200 000
Total	11 000 000	8 800 000	2 200 000

Table 13.4 Programme administration cost vs. cost savings

Programme cost (US$)	Programme savings (US$)	Return on investment (US$)
1 045 000	2 200 000	1 155 000

Determining the costs is only one part of the equation. The more complex task is estimating the savings of the programme – savings occur when the goals are achieved. It is important to track the actual costs versus the benefits on a regular basis. If interim adjustments are required a cost–benefit analysis may allow for these variances. The benefits of bringing a disabled worker back to work are considerable. The cost–benefit analysis can be calculated using only the direct impact on premiums, or broader benefits can be examined such as improved morale of the worker and the workforce, improved productivity, and avoidance of replacement workers and retraining costs. A simple analysis is demonstrated in Table 13.3 and programme administration costs versus cost savings are shown in Table 13.4.

A significant amount of data can be collected and analysed to assist in achieving a smooth-running programme with defendable results.

The results of data analysis must be presented in a format that is appropriate for reviewing and interpreting. To decide on the format an understanding of the organization must be present.

Future costs and benefits

A sophisticated cost analysis includes benefits expected to occur in the future. Successful rehabilitation for disabled employees means that the individual will become productive and not require additional services in the future (Rajkumar & French 1997). Improvements in work skills, psychological adjustment and physical health may have longterm benefits. However, these are hard to estimate as one cannot predict all the future variables. If an attempt is made to estimate potential future savings, a current value of future benefits calculation may well be required as US$100 today has a higher value now than it will in the future – 10 years from now the savings projections will be greater. Whatever the projected future costs and benefits, assumptions must be made. Since there is great latitude in selecting assumptions and making approximations, it is essential that the evaluator openly specify and document the assumptions, and the reasons they were specified (Posavac & Carey 2003). This will assist in replicating the data point in the future and understanding why the evaluator chose to target specific future data indicators but not others while performing the cost–benefit analysis.

Corrective action

One of the true values of measuring outcomes is the ability to adjust the programme in any areas where gaps arise. To ensure ultimate programme success it is essential to develop action plans to close any gaps that are identified during the evaluation phase.

Evaluation of preferred providers

As discussed previously, preferred providers may be used to assist in facilitating care for the injured or ill employee. It is essential that the outcomes of these interventions be measured. It is recommended that performance standards are established at the outset of any preferred provider relationship outlining expectations. Performance standards must be measurable and should be reported on regularly.

Management review – reports

The development and communication of management reports can be one of the essential success elements of the programme. Communication is a multidimensional, interactive process, therefore reports and the communication of results also need to be multidimensional and interactive (Posavac & Carey 2003). Often programme results are not communicated sufficiently, creating questions around the value of programmes in the workplace. Outcome measurement and evaluation is vital to any programme, particularly when a DM programme can have such a broad effect in the workplace and the operation of the business. It is essential that the communication of results is carried out on an aggregate basis so that the identity of those on disability or RTW programmes is not revealed.

It is a good idea to plan the communication schedule and the information that will be conveyed, as demonstrated in Table 13.5.

It is also a good idea to perform an ongoing exploration of communication needs and modify the communication to suit the information requirements of the various stakeholders in the process. Before deciding on the form or the formality of this communication it is good to ask 'What are the needs?' and 'What is the purpose?'. The answers to these questions will clarify the type of reporting that is best suited to the situation.

The two most common forms of communication are written and presentations.

Table 13.5 Plan of the communication schedule

Role	Detail	Type of correspondence	Timeframe
Direct manager	Progress and specific interventions	Memo format Informal meeting	Once a month or as required
Director	Progress updates	Report	Quarterly and annually
Senior management	Progress updates	Report Presentation	Annually or as requested
Employees	Individually per case	Meetings Memos Data results postings	As required
Supervisors	Progress per case Specific interventions	Meetings Memos	As required

Written reports

Written reports provide a formal summary of the results of the programme and may be required periodically to have important evaluation information documented. As discussed in Cooper and Schindler (2003), 'reports have identifiable components'. Written reports will generally follow the outline of executive summary, introduction, body/findings and recommendations/conclusions. The written report can be geared to the audience. Writers must ask themselves 'Who will be reading the report?' and 'Who might it be passed on to?'. The predisposing intent of the report should be explored and the preconceived notion that may be held by the audience must also be understood. A caution in any technical report is to avoid jargon or acronyms that the reader may not be familiar with and struggle to interpret. The base knowledge level should never be assumed. The sections and detail can be cut or added to depending on the needs of the reader.

Title page

The title page provides the title of the report, the author, and the date and company particulars.

Executive summary

The executive summary is an important method of capturing the key recommendations coming from the report. The summary is expected to be concise and to the point. Often senior executives do not have the time or patience to read the entire report so this will help to ensure that the key findings are communicated in a manner that demonstrates, to senior executives, the steps that need to be taken. The executive summary can drive the potential outcomes of the project by ensuring it is clear and brief. Generally, one to two pages of bullet points is acceptable.

Index

The index is of particular importance if the report is going to deal with more than one item.

Introduction

The introduction outlines the purpose of the report and highlights the need for the exploration of an issue being examined. It may summarize the problem statement, the research objectives, the background, and the reason for the synthesis of information or the cause for the report. The introduction should tell the reader what the contents of the report are and cover all the essential topic areas. Nothing should be in the body that is not covered in the introduction.

Methodology

If the report is a research report there should be a section expanding on how the data were handled, what data were collected, the sample design, the research design and the data analysis methods. Any limitations or extraneous variables should be covered here. If the limitations and variables are not discussed it can put into question the findings when readers ask themselves how a certain situation was handled. An example of this is in measuring the decrease in the number of accidents over a given period. If the report is going to demonstrate raw data and the numbers have dramatically reduced – but the report does not indicate that the employee population has decreased by 30% over the same time due to transferring employees to a new facility – the results will be suspect.

Body/findings

This is generally the largest section of the report. It should contain subheadings for ease of reading. It may be useful to split the sections into different pages if the sections are long and/or cumbersome. It is necessary to use sufficient amounts of empty space to encourage readers to wade through a voluminous report. Graphs can be inserted directly into the report, and the data to support the graphs placed in the appendix.

Recommendations/conclusions

A brief statement to reinforce the purpose of the report is required to finalize it. Recommendations and conclusions should not provide any new information. This section is meant to summarize the recommendations and conclusions coming from the report.

Appendix

Back-up data for the report can be appendices in a sequential order from the body of the report. The appendix may vary in length and complexity depending on the audience and the requirement for quick access to the evidence at a later date.

Bibliography

Not all reports will require a bibliography. However, if research or documented literature is used to prove a point or emphasize an issue then proper citations, style and formats need to be used here.

It is important to write the report in draft then read and edit it for accuracy, tone, spelling and grammar. Wherever possible, ownership words like 'I' should be avoided – a report conveys factual information to support a programme or express a proposal on a topic. It is not a personal biography or opinion on an issue. Use of 'I' in reports reduces the business-like tone. Although this sounds like basic advice it is quite interesting how many times reports are composed and sent without a review to catch obvious errors.

Presentations

Personal presentations are a very effective means of communication in our high-tech communication-orientated society. The number of emails and memos managers receive is high and a report delivered in this manner may not get read or addressed in a timely manner. A brief presentation meeting ensures that the information is conveyed and allows the participants an opportunity to discuss results and 'brainstorm' about continuous improvement ideas. Personal presentations are effective as they can be adjusted during the actual presentation based on feedback, and responses areas can be emphasized and expanded upon to address questions.

Presentations can be set up with a short background, summary of results and recommendations, then details around each of the key programme components (including future plans) to enhance the programme, and then the appropriate call for questions from the audience. It is helpful to project the results using an overhead or a computer-aided projection system, and to provide copies of the presentation to the participants for note-taking and something to take away with them to reinforce the findings.

Presentations should follow general presentation rules of not having too much information on the slides and using a variety of methods to convey the information such as pie charts, graphs or tables. One error presenters commonly make is that they suddenly believe everyone has to be able to tell a joke just because they are standing in front of an audience. Jokes should be avoided as they can reduce the seriousness of your message and even harm your reputation. It is interesting how most people can remember the first statement a presenter makes and determine if they will continue to listen or 'tune out' based on it.

It is sometimes advisable to have reviewed the presentation and the desired outcome with a member of the audience in advance so they can provide you with some support should the group start to tune out or seriously question your recommendations. It is also a good idea to draw on a member of the audience for a specific case sample. An example of this would be if you are reporting the results of the modified work programme. You could use one of the managers with a positive outcome as a brief case study to support the implementation of the programme company-wide or to support the continuation of the programme in the following year. It requires speaking with the manager (one of the participants) in advance and discussing the 'comfort level' of the case and his or her willingness to endorse the programme. It makes for great conversation during the presentation.

There are many presentation skills around voice, non-verbal behaviours, distractions and audiovisual aids (such as not putting too much information on slides). Disability management practitioners should acquire a familiarity with these skills and be familiar with presentation techniques prior to presenting to a senior management team.

CONCLUSION

Programme evaluation and the communication of the results is an important component of any DM programme. Disability management practitioners who master these skills assist in securing and maintaining the importance of this practice area within corporations.

REFERENCES

Cooper D R, Schindler P S 2003 Business Research Methods, 8th edn. McGraw-Hill Higher Education, New York, p 660

Posavac J E, Carey R G 2003 Program Evaluation: Methods and case studies, 6th edn. Prentice Hall, New Jersey

Rajkumar A S, French M T 1997 Drug abuse crime costs and the economic benefits of treatment. Journal of Quantitative Criminology 13:291–323

Van Beek G, Kuvaja K 2000 The role of quality management in the European platform for vocational rehabilitation. Disability and Rehabilitation 22(8):379–382

Wholey J S 1983 Evaluation and Effective Public Management. Little, Brown, Boston

Chapter **14**

Communication

LEARNING OBJECTIVES

- Understand the importance of effective communication
- Review the various rehabilitation models
- Review the centrality of disability management to the recovery process

---

INTRODUCTION

Perhaps the most important component of disability management (DM) is effective communication. This chapter will examine the importance of interactions between all of the participants in the DM process and suggest a model for effective communication.

Everyone in the practice of DM is familiar with cases that have gone on for years and which should have ended much earlier. Such cases perplex us and are extremely costly to the individual, the family, the employer and society. Typically these cases 'go off-track' as a result of poor communication throughout the process. In order to better understand what happens, the following case is presented.

Case study   Bill's story

Bill is a 49-year-old factory worker who has been with same employer for 30 years. While coming to the employer with no specific skill set he has worked his way into a millwright position and is now considered a very skilled employee. Like many others, his skills are specific to the type of machinery used and, as he does not have trades qualifications, it would be difficult for him to find employment elsewhere. Given the seniority level and skill level he has attained, his wages plus overtime average approximately US$110 000 a year; in some years he makes substantially more with overtime. His income has allowed him a lifestyle full of 'toys' and a beautiful house on an acreage. There is a mortgage with five years left before it is paid off, and he is making payments on a new truck. His wife is employed at the local college as a secretary and of their three adult children, one lives at home and the two others and their families live close by.

continued overpage

However, Bill has not worked for three years. One day he was replacing an electrical motor in a conveyor system. He was bent over trying to remove the old motor when he felt a searing pain in his lower back and collapsed to the floor. He was attended to by the First Aid officer who called an ambulance and Bill was taken to the local hospital. At the hospital Bill was in pain and confused. He was taken to the ER but treatment was delayed as the emergency personnel could not immediately get information from him. Eventually he was treated with painkillers and a muscle relaxant and was kept in for observation overnight. He was released into the care of his physician the next day. His physician told him that he had severely strained his lower back and that he would like to proceed with conservative treatment. The physician – the medical treatment provider (MTP) – continued with painkillers and a muscle relaxant and told Bill to stay off work for three weeks. After this time Bill was still in pain and the physician told him to stay home for another three weeks. Bill was still having difficulty so the physician booked him for a computed tomography (CT) scan and kept him off work until the scan could be completed. It took three months before Bill had the scan. During all this time his employer was not contacted and only received the paperwork through the Workers' Compensation Board (WCB). The CT scan showed a very slight disc herniation at L5–S1 and the physician suggested non-invasive treatment, which consisted of medication and a statement to stay as active as possible. However, he suggested that Bill stay off work for another six weeks.

Eventually, out of sheer boredom, Bill became more active doing chores around the house. One day he was lifting some laundry when he again had a severe pain in his lower back, collapsed to the floor and could not straighten up for several hours. When he went to his physician he was simply referred to an orthopaedic surgeon. He was able to see the surgeon two months later, who ordered another CT scan and a magnetic resonance imaging (MRI) scan. He explained that the CT scan had a waiting list of two months and the MRI one of 13 months. He would only go ahead with the MRI if the CT was inclusive, which unfortunately it was. After waiting in great pain for over a year Bill finally had the MRI and saw the surgeon shortly afterwards. The MRI confirmed the herniation and that it was not retracting; the surgeon suggested surgery. Bill agreed and he was put on the waiting list. Six weeks later he underwent the surgery. His recovery was difficult – he had some immediate pain relief but was soon complaining about the same pain and leg weakness as before. The surgeon told him that the surgery had been a complete success but that he possibly had some scar tissue forming which was causing the ongoing problems. The surgeon suggested that if it did not improve Bill may have to undergo further surgery. Needless to say Bill was not thrilled by this prospect. His insurer suggested a rehabilitation programme at a local clinic and Bill agreed to go.

Since then Bill has undergone various rehabilitation programmes but has not gone back to work. Now, after several failed rehabilitation programmes, the insurer has decided that Bill is fit to return to work (RTW) and is planning on ending his benefits in two weeks. The employer will not take him back since he is not fit for duties and the family physician is at a loss as to what to do. For the first time in his life Bill is looking at being unemployed.

What went wrong?

In a non-workplace injury or illness most recovery processes would operate in a way similar to Figure 14.1.

The problem with expectations

The entire process would unfold as in normal timeframes and the workers would RTW or to normal activities as soon as they were able. In an insurance environment this normal process becomes more complicated and prone to delays as a result of the introduction of more complex expectations. In the

Figure 14.1 Example of a recovery process in non-workplace injury or illness.

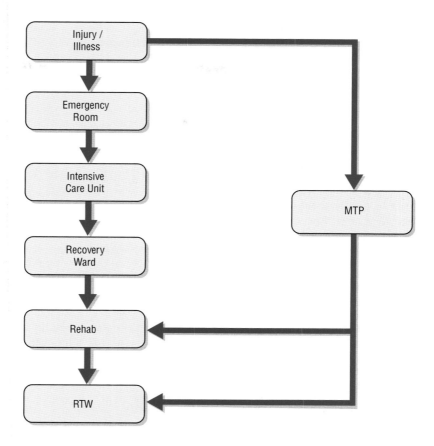

normal process the workers expect to be treated, as under the norms of their systems, expect to recover and to get on with their lives. Their families interact with them, and by and large the goal is to recover and move on with life. In an insurance environment, while all the preceding expectations also exist, other expectations are added, such as:

- being paid
- receiving special assistance such as home care or maid service
- job security
- possible retraining into another job
- receiving a large financial settlement.

In some cases these expectations can be negative, such as expecting to be poorly treated or taken advantage of by the insurance company. If the employer has a poor record of accommodating workers returning post-injury this may also lead to negative expectations. Such negative expectations can result in a worker being reluctant to cooperate in the RTW process.

In the first three stages of this process the expectations are probably universal. The person expects to be medically well cared for and that their needs (and the needs of the family) are taken care of. This assurance is critical to the recovery process. Once the person is past the immediate danger he or she expects:

continued overpage

- to be well-treated and well-informed by the medical community
- to hear from the insurance company
- to hear from the employer
- to hear from friends and colleagues/workmates
- to be told what is going to happen.

These expectations are very reasonable and when they are met they aid in the workers' recovery. If they are not met, doubts begin to form. If workers are not well-treated or well-informed by the physician, for example, they will begin to wonder if all is well or if they should be more worried about their condition. If they do not hear from the insurance company they will begin to wonder about their benefits and about how the bills will get paid and how the family will get fed. If they do not hear from the employer they will begin to wonder about the status of their employment and whether or not they will be welcomed back. If they do not hear from friends and colleagues they will begin to wonder if they are valued and may begin to think that something else is happening. If they are not told what is going to happen they start thinking of the worst-case scenario and begin entertaining very negative thoughts at a time when they should be positively focused.

In Bill's case he was in and out of hospital quickly. His expectations of being treated well were probably met, though things would have progressed more smoothly if someone from his workplace had gone with him to the hospital; they then could have answered the hospital's questions so that treatment could have commenced sooner. Bill's physician accepted the diagnosis provided by the hospital and did not follow suggested guidelines for the treatment of a low back strain which included immediate activity. He also does not explain to Bill what has happened to him, how long recovery is expected to take and when he can expect to return to work. As a result, Bill has no idea what to expect – he does not know when he should expect to start to feel better and what he should do to help himself. In the absence of this information he will form his own conclusions, which, typically, are negative.

Staying at home, Bill begins to feel isolated. He has had no contact from his employer, other than right at the beginning when he received a phone call to ensure that he had filled out his forms. The only contact with the insurer has been a letter informing him that his claim has been accepted and what the amount of his cheque would be. Initially, friends and workmates visited or called but that dropped off. The longer he is at home, the less contact Bill has with the workplace and the outside world in general. Eventually he begins to wonder if anyone cares about him at all. Specifically, related to employment he begins to wonder if his employer cares about him, values him and wants him back. In the absence of direct confirmation to the contrary he will assume that the employer does not care and does not want him back.

At this stage simple contact from the insurer and the employer could avoid many subsequent problems. This is the opportune time to ensure that Bill feels like a valued human being and employee. Regular contact with his workmates and phone calls from his supervisor, for example, would ensure that he stays connected with his worksite and keeps himself orientated toward work, and therefore his self-esteem would remain intact.

In the absence of information and in the face of abject boredom, Bill begins to become more active. However, as a result of not being informed, he begins with activity that allows him to exacerbate his injury. Had he received information or had he been referred for rehabilitative treatment he would have been exposed to education and exercise appropriate to his condition and the disc herniation may never have occurred.

Nevertheless, the herniation does occur. The orthopaedic surgeon supplies Bill with a little more information but Bill goes into the surgery relatively uninformed and unaware of the all-too-common risk of scar tissue. He is left alone during all this time and during his recovery. He is allowed to draw his own conclusions.

Communication finally occurs when the insurer informs Bill that he is being sent to a rehabilitation clinic for treatment. He is informed that the goal of the treatment is to get him back to work. Bill is upset because his goal is to be pain-free again. Bill goes to the clinic where he meets young and enthusiastic occupational therapists (OTs), kinesiologists (KINs) and physiotherapists (PTs). They extol the virtues of exercise and get Bill going on an exercise programme. No one discusses the mismatch of his expectation (to be pain-free) and their expectation (that he RTW). As a result, after Bill has spent a few weeks exercising in pain, he refuses to continue and is discharged for non-compliance. Now the communication with the insurer begins and threatens to terminate Bill's benefits if he does not cooperate in treatment. Bill's expectation of his insurance company – that it is there to help him and fund his recovery – begins to change and he becomes wary. The insurer asks him to return to his physician who is sympathetic to Bill's complaints of pain but who also wants Bill to return to the rehabilitation clinic.

Bill is referred to a different clinic which includes an educational component in the treatment regimen. Bill learns what has happened to him and, for the first time, can discuss his sense of isolation, his fears about recovery and going back to work, and the losses he has experienced due to his post-surgical condition. He does better in the programme and is ready to attempt to RTW.

For the first time in nearly three years the employer is contacted by the insurer in an effort to RTW. All previous communication had been in writing and only involved information regarding costs. Now the employer, who has assumed that Bill was never coming back, is amazed to hear that they are to take him back. Understandably, they are reluctant and insist on medical evidence that Bill is 'safe' to come back. They insist that Bill needs to be able to perform 100% of his duties before they will consider taking him back. When Bill hears this he is furious. He has given 30 years of his life to this company and now they are throwing him aside. He quickly begins to deteriorate and his physician, concerned about the increase in Bill's pain level, states in writing that Bill needs more time and that the RTW should be delayed for another six weeks.

The insurer has had enough and considers that this latest doctor's note is a stalling ploy and is ready to deem Bill as able to RTW. If Bill is unwilling to do so they will terminate his benefits and he will be without an income.

Everyone in the practice of DM knows that this case is very unlikely to come to a happy conclusion and that, as bad as it is, it could have been even worse. There could have been multiple surgeries, drug dependency, familial break-up and much more. How would this have been different with more effective communication?

WHAT SHOULD HAVE HAPPENED?

With truly effective communication Bill would have heard from both his employer and his insurer very early in the process. The insurer would have explained how the benefits work, what is expected of Bill and that the goal of treatment is both physical recovery and RTW. The employer would have informed Bill of their DM programme and how they would assist him once he was ready to RTW. They also would have outlined a regular communication strategy, letting Bill know that they would be in regular contact just checking on how he is doing and seeing if there was anything they could do to help. This contact would have continued as long as he was away from work.

The physician would have informed Bill about the nature of a back strain, the symptoms, length of expected recovery, possible difficulties and, after

Bill's recovery was extended, he would have referred him to physiotherapy or to an exercise programme. The orthopaedic surgeon would have informed Bill more clearly on the risks of surgery and in particular the frequency of difficulties with scar tissue. He would have informed Bill that conservative treatment might still have been an option.

The clinicians in the rehabilitation clinic would have taken time to help Bill deal with some of his emotional issues and would have recognized and dealt with his pain issues as was eventually done in the second clinic. Finally, if this had all been done there would have been no surprise at the end of the process. In fact, quite possibly the strain would have resolved itself and Bill may have returned to work at that point.

Most critically to all of the above is the need to identify and address expectations. Many times we do not state our expectations but we do have them, then when they are not met we react. Given the lack of attention to Bill, he was never given the opportunity to state his expectations, nor was the employer, nor was the insurer. Everything was just assumed; assumptions are very dangerous. With excellent communication skills time and energy go into making all expectations overt so that no assumptions are made and all expectations can be addressed.

MODELS OF COMMUNICATION

Pransky et al (2004), after conducting an extensive literature review, identify four models of communication common in the field of DM:

1. The medical model.
2. The physical rehabilitation model.
3. The job-match model.
4. The managed care model.

They argue that while the DM process seeks to incorporate elements of each of these models, eventually one emerges as the predominant model.

THE MEDICAL MODEL

The medical model places the MTP at its centre. This model can be termed 'the traditional model' and is the model favoured by insurance providers. In this model not only does the medical treatment provider physically treat the person, he or she also provide opinions on the suitability of certain types of work for the individual. This despite that fact that they have little or no knowledge of what that work requires. Communication in this model is usually unidirectional with all information emanating from the MTP.

In relatively simple cases, such as strains, sprains, etc., this model can be quite effective. However, when certain complications arise, such as mental health disorders or when conditions become chronic, this model begins to break down. Most MTPs do not have the expertise to deal with these conditions, nor are they compensated for taking the time to learn about work conditions even if they are inclined to do so. This model is based entirely on the expertise of the MTP. The opinions and perspectives of patients or employers are rarely taken into consideration. This model has frequently pitted MTPs against insurers and employers. One result of this has been that the MTP is viewed with suspicion by these groups and is often referred to and discounted as a 'patient advocate', which in this context denotes keeping the person away from work contrary to what the objective evidence may say based solely on the subjective evidence presented by the patient. In the cases typically dealt with in the DM process this model has proven to be highly ineffective and problematic, frequently leading to confrontation and rarely to solutions.

Positive points about this model are:

- works well in basic cases of simple musculoskeletal injuries
- the physician is often respected by the client, who may follow treatment suggestions.

Negative points about the model are:

- communication is unidirectional
- physicians know very little about the workplace
- physicians have no incentives to become better informed
- works poorly with chronic injuries
- cannot deal with psychosocial issues
- short visits make it hard to determine what is really going on.

THE PHYSICAL REHABILITATION MODEL

Similar to the medical model, in many ways this model is also primarily unidirectional in its orientation. Based primarily in rehabilitation treatment facilities, PTs, OTs and KINs focus on restoring the person's functional abilities so that they can RTW. Even when the programmes include a focus on psychosocial issues the ultimate goal is to provide enough reassurance so that the person will at least attempt to RTW. Further, the focus is primarily on fitting the worker to the job rather than the job to the worker. This is not a desired outcome of DM. In favour of this model, the professionals involved are often viewed to have more credibility than that of the physician, employer or insurer. They often work with the person on a daily basis for six weeks or longer and are much more able to comment on the person's progress and mental state than is the physician. Nevertheless, this model is no better at addressing the very complex issues than is the medical model.

Positive points about this model are:

- the person is seen over a longer period of time
- focus on restoring function
- very pragmatically orientated
- more awareness and knowledge of the worksite.

Negative points about this model are:

- communication is unilateral
- psychosocial issues are often identified but not treated
- information from the worksite is often dismissed as being subjective and therefore of no use
- treatment programmes are based on unproven assumptions.

THE JOB-MATCH MODEL

This model strives to fit people with functional impairments into a specific job that is suitable to someone with those impairments. In doing so many types of tests and measures are used on both the individual and the job. This model assumes that both the restrictions of the worker and the requirements of the job are easily and accurately quantifiable. But this is simply not the case. As with the other two models mentioned above, this model ignores psychosocial factors when matching worker to job, which is a factor that is more than likely going to lead to failure. Another feature of this model is that those practising it have a tendency to believe that it is an accurate science. Thus their reports tend to read like pronouncements, trying to emulate medicolegal reports when in fact key elements, such as worksite conditions, personal interactions and 'subjective' opinions of the supervisor, for example, have been ignored or discounted. In fact, such 'subjective' opinions are critical and often more accurate than all the tests and measures as they are based on the reality of the worksite, not some model derived in the pristine setting of a laboratory or clinic.

A positive point about this model is the collection of data regarding job functions.

Negative points about this model are:

- communication is unilateral
- it does not address psychosocial factors
- based on questionable science.

THE MANAGED CARE MODEL

This model assumes that by setting certain parameters around disability duration and then managing people and the system more vigorously, people will RTW more quickly. The parameters or norms are established based on data from workers' compensation, insurance and population health analysts. These data are then used to form certain 'bands' of expectation for recovery and RTW. If a worker exceeds a band then intensive intervention is indicated. Two key assumptions in this model are that delays are primarily caused by administrative bottlenecks or by lack of motivation in the worker. Based on these assumptions case management interventions are used to eliminate delays and motivate the worker.

Positive points about this model are:

- provides a framework against which to measure progress
- identifies administrative delays
- provides focus for limited resources.

Negative points about this model are:

- no early intervention
- focuses on delayed cases
- often blames workers for delays.

Summary

In all of the models presented above communication is unidirectional. All of the models seek to focus communication on the needs of one system or another. Pransky et al (2004: 626–627) state that 'although a particular disability-prevention process may incorporate elements of several models, most bear a predominant resemblance to one of these four stereotypes'. If this is indeed the case it is unfortunate. This conclusion requires that DM be subsumed by something else. This is in fact not the case. Disability management is the process. It is not subsumed in any of these models. It requires its own model.

THE COMPREHENSIVE DISABILITY MANAGEMENT MODEL

In this communication model, communication is multidirectional and the DM provider is the centre of the model. In comprehensive disability management (CDM) neither the MTP nor the OT, PT or KIN are left in charge of the process. All are valuable members of the team and all have valuable opinions that can be used in the process. However, the DM practitioner ensures that this information is acquired in a timely manner and at the appropriate stage of the process. Opinions are sought when needed and provided to the correct person in the process. Whether that is the insurance professional, the physician or the employer, the DM practitioner ensures that they acquire the information that they need when they need it.

A key component in this process is to make sure that all expectations from all parties involved are clearly identified. Hidden expectations or unstated assumptions must be made overt and clearly identified. This allows everyone to know what to expect and when to expect it as well as knowing how progress will be measured. An effective communication process will ensure that there are no surprises for anyone.

Most importantly the DM practitioner ensures that the person with the disability is kept informed throughout the process. The injured or ill person is the key component in the system. Supposedly all the systems and all the professionals are involved in order to help the person recover and RTW or to normal daily activities. They are not there to serve the interests of the system they represent, though this is often forgotten. The DM practitioner ensures that the focus stays on the person, to the benefit of the system.

In order to do this the DM practitioner must interact with all the professionals involved in the system. Consequently they must be familiar with the stereotypical models of communication. However, familiarity does not imply an adoption of these systems. For example, if information is required from a physician the practitioner must know the best way of acquiring this information. This requires being familiar with how physicians and their offices function; it does not require functioning in the same manner. Similarly, information from the rehabilitation professional or from job-bank data may be required. Again, this means that the practitioner must know how to get that information. They must enter those communication models and acquire what is needed but not become part of that model. The focus must always be on communicating in such a way as to do what is best for the individual.

This may sound like advocacy and in a way it is. Remember that we began with a stated assumption that work is a necessary and desired part of all our lives. Given this assumption, what is best for a person is to be able to participate fully in the workforce. This is what the DM practitioner is advocating for and this must be made clear to the client at the beginning of the process. Thus the needs of the person, the needs of the employer and the needs of society merge in one desired outcome: to enable the person to recover and RTW as soon as is appropriate.

The CDM model of communication is demonstrated in Figure 14.2.

In a CDM model the DM practitioner is involved from the time of injury or illness. They ensure that all expectations are identified; they also ensure that all forms are filled out so that there are no delays in insurance payments. The practitioner monitors the care that the person is receiving and ensures that there are no administrative bureaucratic delays. The

Figure 14.2 Comprehensive disability management model of communication.

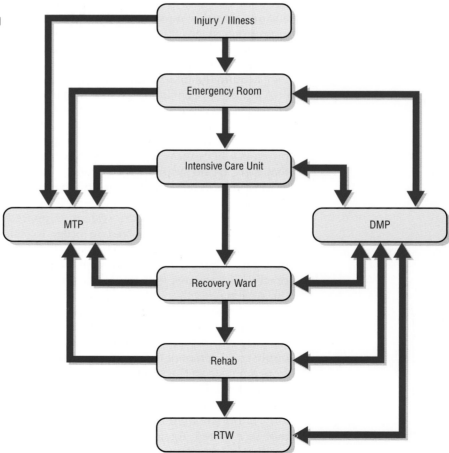

practitioner makes sure the employer is aware of what is happening and, when timely, provides the physician with accurate worksite information. If there are questions regarding eligibility for benefits or the nature of benefits the practitioner identifies the issues and determines the answers. The practitioner keeps the employer informed of all developments and readies the workplace to take the person. If psychosocial issues are identified, the practitioner arranges for appropriate professionals to assist in resolving these issues. In short, the DM practitioner is at the centre of the process and ensures that all communication is occurring effectively in all directions.

CONCLUSION

How would Bill's case have unfolded if a DM practitioner had been involved?

A worksite with a CDM programme would have had someone go to the hospital with Bill and would have provided the ER triage nurse with the information required. As soon as appropriate the practitioner would have met Bill and perhaps his family to explain the process, clarify expectations and outline a schedule of events and key communication points. This meeting would not be a surprise as Bill would have received education regarding the CDM programme during education sessions at work. The practitioner would also receive Bill's consent to be able to see the information necessary to begin planning Bill's return to work. Based on best-practice guidelines the practitioner would monitor Bill's progress and ensure that everything was happening as it should. He or she would encourage Bill to stay in touch with his employer and his colleagues, to keep Bill connected with his workmates and to remind him that he is an important part of the team.

If treatment is not progressing as per clinical guidelines, the practitioner may meet the MTP to clarify the situation and suggest resources available through the employer or with which the MTP may not be familiar. In Bill's case this may have meant referral to a clinic or PT before he herniated his disc. In this case that did not happen. Post-herniation, the DM practitioner would provide Bill with any information about surgical outcomes, or other information pertinent to spinal surgery that would help him be an informed consumer of these medical services. The practitioner would have let the employer know that RTW was being delayed due to the surgery and would have provided the employer with a new estimated RTW date. Most critically, during Bill's treatment in the rehabilitation clinics, the practitioner would have assured effective communication by making all expectations explicit, thereby avoiding misunderstandings and unnecessary frustrations.

In our scenario Bill does not RTW. It is quite conceivable that effective communication as outlined above would have led to an entirely different result and avoided the pain and suffering inherent in such a situation.

Effective communication is the most important tool in CDM. As Amick et al (2000) showed, more open, receptive communication by employers led to more positive RTW outcomes.

REFERENCES

Amick B, Habeck R V, Hunt A et al 2000 Measuring the impact of organizational behaviors on work disability prevention and management. Journal of Occupational Rehabilitation 10(1):21–38

Pransky G S, Shaw W S, Franche R L et al 2004 Disability prevention and communication among workers, physicians, employers, and insurers – current models and opportunities for improvement. Disability and Rehabilitation 26(11):625–634

Chapter **15**

Ethics in disability management

LEARNING OBJECTIVES

■ To be able to define ethical behaviour
■ Understand the need for ethics in disability management
■ Review the origins of the formulation of ethics

INTRODUCTION

In our society today the word 'ethics' is frequently heard in the media. For example, politicians are often accused of unethical behaviour, there are ethics commissioners and codes of ethics of various kinds but what is actually meant when we use the term 'ethics'? Is there a common understanding that allows us to clearly understand what is meant when ethical behaviour is discussed? This chapter will provide a general overview of what comprises the study of ethics, the theory of ethics and several ethical codes as well as a decision-making process for when one is confronted with having to make an ethical decision.

WHAT ARE ETHICS?

Very simply, ethics are the factors on which we base the decisions on how we should lead our lives and the determinants of why we make the decisions we do. Ethics help guide us through difficult and complex situations, and also affect the most basic of decisions. For example, should I steal the chocolate bar when no one is looking; or should I turn in the wallet I found in the hallway; or should I withdraw life support from an ailing parent. All of these are ethical questions of varying complexity. How does one decide what to do? At the very simple level the response may be to do what is right. But how does one determine what is right and what is wrong? One person or culture may view an action as wrong while another may view it as right. How do we then determine what are right or wrong actions?

In professions, unethical practice can lead to serious repercussions up to including the loss of the ability to practise one's profession. What distinguishes a professional body from others is the existence and enforcement of a code of ethics, sometimes also referred to as a code of practice or code of conduct. Members of the profession agree to function according to this code and to be disciplined if they transgress it. Therefore, ethics and the subsequent ethical behaviour is a defining factor in the practice of a profession. But how is such a code derived and why is it needed?

WHY DO WE NEED ETHICS?

When we are faced with a dilemma over which action to take, ethics enable us to determine the most correct course of action. A professional, when faced with such a dilemma, consults the code of ethics of that profession and makes a decision based on that code. Professionals may consult others within their profession, or ethical experts, in the process of making the decision but the code of ethics remains the central and deciding factor in the decision. Thus ethics informs us as to what to do.

Ethics allow for the protection of one's self and the client. For the most part codes of ethics fall into two categories: aspirational and enforceable. Aspirational codes have lofty goals that state how a people should conduct themselves. These codes simply state the things that we aspire to, not what we have to do or not do. This is the territory of enforceable codes that have the ability to punish anyone who transgresses the code. For example, an aspirational ethical statement may be something to the effect that all professionals will strive to treat their clients with dignity and respect. If challenged it is always possible to argue that one was striving at the limit of one's ability even though one was found lacking. An enforceable code would say that all professionals will treat their clients with dignity and respect, and add subsections which specify how dignity and respect are manifested in the professional–client relationship. This information is made public and a client can then determine if a professional has, in their opinion, acted unethically. They can then bring a complaint against the professional to the professional body which can investigate and determine if the professional has indeed violated the code and acted unethically. This ability affords the public some measure of protection from any unethical behaviour of professionals.

This agreed-upon code of ethics then is a standard of measure against which the actions of a professional can be measured. If in the situation outlined above, the professional attempts a defence, the code of ethics allows for a basis on which the behaviour can be judged. In essence, the ethics of the profession become the basic laws of the profession to the extent that cases can be (and often are) taken before the courts to resolve. Given the importance of such a process to the protection of the consumers of a professional service and the dire consequences that can result if a professional is found in violation of an ethical principle it would seem of great importance that everyone agrees on these principles and, in essence, agrees on what constitutes right and wrong behaviour.

HOW DO WE DECIDE WHAT IS RIGHT AND WRONG?

Over time, various ethical theories have been developed. What follows is a brief discussion of the major theories.

Cultural relativism

Cultural relativism is an argument against the universality of ethical theories. It argues that:

- different societies have different moral codes
- there is no objective or universal truth in ethics or morals
- therefore, what is determined to be moral is solely determined by one's own culture.

There are several problems with this argument. If it is correct then we have no right to criticize or challenge other cultures or even our own. For example, we as a society encourage people to question other countries' beliefs and practices. North Korea and China are frequently being chastised for their human rights violations. However, if cultural relativism is correct then we have no right to criticize or punish these countries for not changing their practices. We simply have to accept that their ethical understanding is different to ours.

Cultural relativism argues that there are no universal truths in ethics or morals. Yet there appear to be some universal moral or ethical rules that are accepted across societies and cultures. For example, lying and murder do not appear to be acceptable behaviour in any culture.

Cultural relativism also implies that our own culture is perfect and that no moral progress is necessary or can be made. It does not allow us to judge previous standards in our own time – we must judge them in the time that they were made because they were morally just in that time period and to say that they are better now is the kind of judgement that cultural relativism says we cannot make. For example, polygamy was acceptable in an earlier time but now society believes that it is completely unacceptable regardless of religious beliefs. However, if you believe cultural relativism it is not possible to make that judgement.

Lastly and perhaps most problematical, cultural relativism argues that moral progress or cultural reform, as we define it, cannot be made since the ideals of society at any given point are correct and therefore do not need to change. Therefore, given this theory, apartheid in South Africa should have been left to function unchallenged by the rest of the world as South Africa deemed it to be culturally appropriate at the time. However, this was not the case since the world punished South Africa for its use of apartheid.

Ethical subjectivism

Ethical subjectivism is a theory that expounds on the nature of moral judgements. There are two ethical theories in this category: simple subjectivism and emotivism.

Simple subjectivism

Simple subjectivism states that moral opinions are based on our feelings and if they are sincere then they cannot be wrong. Put simply, if X is good or right then you approve of X, but if X is bad or wrong then you disapprove of X.

A counterpoint to simple subjectivism is the infallibility argument. This logic proceeds as follows: if one is speaking honestly or sincerely then one's moral judgements cannot be mistaken. However, one may be mistaken in one's moral judgements even if one is speaking sincerely. Therefore, simple subjectivism cannot be true. Take again the example of apartheid. According to simple subjectivism, if one honestly believes that apartheid is right then it is morally right. However, apartheid is morally wrong. Therefore, simple subjectivism is incorrect.

There is another problem with simple subjectivism. Feelings are neither right nor wrong, they simply are. Therefore, there cannot be a disagreement in your moral judgements which are based on your feelings, because feelings cannot be wrong.

Emotivism

Emotivism differs from simple subjectivism in that it takes matters a step further. Not only does one express a feeling but now one also attempts to influence others' behaviours based on this feeling. The logic is as follows: if Y is right (based on an emotional reaction) then do Y. If Y is wrong (based on an emotional reaction) then don't do Y. This appears to be enticingly simple. So what's wrong with this theory?

A major problem with emotivism is that it will allow *any* reason or fact to influence a moral judgement. For example, you have a negative emotional reaction to person Z and decide that you don't like them and that therefore they are bad. I am your friend and you want to convince me that person Z is bad. You also know that person Z is a liberal and, based on previous emotional reactions, I hate liberals. Then all you would have to do is tell me that person Z is a liberal and according to emotivism that is enough for me to decide that person Z is bad. I have judged them before I even meet them or get to know them. It is a small step from this example to concluding that all liberals are bad and something should be done about liberals. Thus emotivism can become a tool for racism and other hate-based attempts to control behaviour and modify ethics.

Religion

The most common place we get or view of morality is through the church and our view of God. By saying this, the authors are not advocating a Judaeo-Christian view of morality. We are simply pointing out that Western societies' views of morality and therefore ethics are irrevocably intertwined with religion and that what are identified as secular views today are in fact based on the religious views of the past.

When examining the influence of religion on ethics there are two theories that must be highlighted. These are the divine command theory and the natural law theory.

The divine command theory

The divine command theory states that:

- If an act is morally right then it is commanded by God.
- If an act is morally wrong then it is forbidden by God.

However, there are many problems associated with this theory such as:

- For this theory to be valid one must first believe in God and if one does not believe in God then this theory does not apply.
- The moral commands are arbitrary. For example, God could have commanded us to lie and then lying would be considered to be good.

A positive aspect of this theory is that it shows how one is held accountable for their actions. For example, there are the Ten Commandments. If one does not follow them, one could go to Hell. These are extremely objective: there is clearly a right and wrong. In modern terms this is an enforceable code.

The natural law theory

The natural law theory states that:

- Everything in nature has a purpose.
- What is morally right is what nature intended. For example, it rains to water the grass and plants. Animals then eat the grass and plants in order to grow and be healthy. Then in turn we kill and eat the animals for us to grow and be healthy. Therefore it is morally acceptable to eat animals.

There are also problems associated with this theory, such as:

- This theory oversimplifies matters. Things do not exist for a single purpose. It is an artificial hierarchal structure that places humans at the top and says that everything is there to support us. In fact, it does not rain in order to feed us. There is a scientific reason for rain and it has nothing to do with watering grass.
- Just because things are natural does not mean it is what it should be or ought to be. The Catholic Church argues that sex is only for procreation and all other forms of sexual behaviour are immoral. Society as a whole does not agree. Another example is that death is a natural consequence of living yet we strive to prolong life as much as possible.
- In order for one to determine what is moral one would have to use one's conscience and reason. Then the moral action taken would be the one with the most or best reason on its side. If this were the case then one's conscience would be the determining factor in making moral decisions. As everyone's conscience differs we would have individual ideas of what is moral and immoral. There would be no agreement on what constitutes moral and ethical behaviour.

Ethical decision-making

The two most popular or well-known processes of ethical decision-making are teleological and deontological (Mattison 2000):

Teleological decision-making

Teleological decision-making – which is also described as consequentialist – looks *only* at the *consequences* of the action at the time the action is judged. The ethical theory that embodies this type of ethical decision-making is utilitarianism.

The theory of utilitarianism has three main parts:

1. *Consequentialism* This states that the right acts are those that maximize good consequences and minimize the bad.
2. *Hedonism* This states that there is only one ultimate good: pleasure or the absence of pain.
3. *Doctrine of impartiality* This states that no one's good or pleasure is to count as more important than anyone else's. Take, for example, the argument over lowering the speed limit of vehicles to prevent accidents and deaths. To determine if lowering the speed limit is a moral action one would have to look at both the positive and negative consequences of the act. One would need to consider, for example, how many people would be saved and how many would be hurt by lowering the speed. If the number of people saved outweighed the number that would be hurt then the moral action would be to lower the speed limit. In fact, it would be immoral not to do so.

There are several problems with this theory. For example:

- Utilitarianism does not take into account the importance of individual rights. For example, you could falsely accuse someone of a crime if doing so will prevent the suffering of a large group of people.
- Utilitarianism suffers from backward-looking logic. For example, you promised a friend you would go out for coffee but you don't really want to go. You would rather stay at home and finish some work, so you don't go. According to utilitarianism it is totally justifiable to break the promise because the work you are doing will benefit more people.
- Utilitarianism is too demanding. It does not distinguish between obligatory actions, which are morally required, from supererogatory actions, which are praiseworthy but not morally required. For example, utilitarianism says that you should not buy new clothes, a car or TV because that money should be used to help those less fortunate than yourself.
- Society does not agree that pleasure is the only ultimate good. Take, for example, the Noziak Experience Machine. Noziak (1974) argued that if pleasure were our only value then 'hooking up' to a pleasure machine for the rest of one's life would be the ultimate human experience. According to utilitarianism, and hedonism in particular, this would be the best choice possible. However, most people would not agree or may even be repulsed by the idea of being hooked up to a machine for pleasure. Thus the claims of hedonism cannot be supported.

Deontological decision-making

Deontological decision-making looks *only* at the *action* itself regardless of the consequences. The ethical theory that embodies this type of decision-making is Kant's ethics. Kant (1959) believed in absolute moral rules, which have no exceptions and must be followed at all times.

Kant had two versions of ethical decision-making: the basic categorical imperative and, later, in an effort to try to deal with the criticisms of this model, he added 'How to treat humans' to the categorical imperative. In Kant's model the main concept of how to determine moral actions is the categorical imperative. This states that an act should *only* be followed *if and only if* one can wish it to become a *universal law*. Therefore, a moral act is when you can wish everyone to follow it, and an immoral act is when a person makes an exception to the rule for oneself. It is to act in a way that you do not want everyone else acting.

Kant developed two types of duties:

1. *Absolute or perfect duties* These are duties that must be followed all the time because they fail the categorical imperative test. Lying and murder are examples of an absolute duty.
2. *Imperfect duty* This duty is one that ought not to be ignored but does not have to be followed. For example, choosing not to help someone even if you are able to. It is possible to live in a world where no one helps anyone else but one would not want to since you may require help at any given time.

There are problems with this theory, such as:

- It gives silly answers to non-moral questions or maxims. For example, I will sell a product such as chocolate but never buy it. It is inconceivable to have a world were everyone sells chocolate but no one buys it. Therefore this action is immoral.
- It gives wrong answers to moral maxims. The categorical imperative tells us that lying is always wrong. However, many of us believe that lying is morally permissible, even required in some cases. For example, there is the commonly cited Inquiring Murderer Case (Kant 1949). A man approaches you and asks if your neighbour is at home. You know that your neighbour is at home. You ask the man why he wants to know and he responds that he intends to kill your neighbour. What do you do? Kant believes that you must tell the truth regardless of the consequence because your perfect duty is to tell the truth not to save the man's life, which is an imperfect duty.
- The categorical imperative fails to give guidance on what maxim one should choose. In the Inquiring Murderer Case there are two maxims: the first is 'I will lie', the second is 'I will save lives'. According to the theory both are perfect duties. How does one choose between them?

Kant eventually developed another version of the categorical imperative in order to deal with the latter criticism. In this theory he stated that one must always treat humanity as an *end* never as a *means* only. An *end* is a *rational being*, which is capable of making his or her own decisions and setting goals. This ability gives an end intrinsic worth. To be treated as an end is to be treated with respect and dignity, someone who is capable of his or her own thought. A *mean*, on the other hand, is a *thing* that is not capable of making its own decisions or setting goals. Means only receive value because humans give it to them. Kant himself perceived a problem with this version in that it would no longer allow for experiments on humans. In order for medical and other experiments to be conducted on humans Kant clarified his means/ends distinction. He stated that it is possible to treat people as a mean if and only if you allow them to give consent or the choice to be used as a mean. By giving them the choice you treat them as both a mean and an end.

It is not hard to see the problems with this theory. For example:

- Requiring that every human be treated as an end seems wrong, especially when it is clear that the person you are treating as an end will treat others as a mean only.
- The division of rational beings and things is too simple. Some non-rational beings deserve the protection of morality as well. For example, society has decided that animals deserve protection.
- There are some non-rational human beings. Kant does not account for them in his virtue theory so are they protected?

One last theory should be mentioned briefly as it appears that the majority of professional ethical codes seem to be based on the virtue theory (Botes 2000). The virtue theory is a relatively simple theory although it has many problems. A virtue theorist asks what traits make a good person. These traits then are those that correspond with virtues. What follows is that a moral person is a person who lives according those virtues.

The dictionary defines a virtue as a particularly efficacious, good or beneficial quality. Examples of virtues are courage, generosity, honesty, kindness and patience. But who picks the virtues? In some cultures the warrior is most virtuous; in others it is the peacemaker. How does one decide who to emulate?

It is also possible for virtues to conflict. For example, if an obese friend asks if they are overweight you must follow the virtue of being honest and tell them 'Yes'. However, by doing so you are being unkind if you answer honestly.

The question remains: what virtue do you follow? The virtue theory does not give any guidance in a situation like that mentioned above. One would have to rely on another ethical theory to come to a conclusion.

PROFESSIONAL ETHICS CODES

Most professions and all health professions have a code of ethics which provides guidance on how to behave in general and more specifically how to interact with clients. Many of these ethical codes are based on virtues or principles that the members are expected to uphold. Four main principles seem to surface when examining these codes. These are:

1. *Autonomy* Informed consent.
2. *Non-malfeasance* To do no harm.
3. *Beneficence* To do what is good for the patient or client.
4. *Justice* The just and fair distribution of goods and services regardless of race, religion, gender, etc. (Hermeren 1999, Huycke & All 2000).

In some professions a fifth principle – responsibility to society – is added. The reasoning for this is because sometimes the action that a professional takes can have a negative effect on more than the individual client, and consideration of such an impact must be taken into account when faced with an ethical dilemma. Even though the virtue theory has many limitations it does allow the individual to apply his or her own ethical principles in making a decision. It does this because the virtues are broad guidelines and do not provide guidance on how to apply them and this allows individuals to provide their own ethical analyses to situations.

HOW DOES ONE MAKE A DECISION?

Many professions include an ethical decision-making model as a companion piece for their code of ethics. This is meant to assist the professional in making a decision when facing an ethical dilemma. Most of these models suggest a step-wise progression in working out the dilemma. When confronting an ethical dilemma, at a minimum the following steps should be considered:

1. If you become aware of an ethical dilemma or potential ethical violation do not become defensive. Keep an open mind.
2. Examine the consequences of the ethical dilemma on everyone who will be affected by it. Consider the situation from all perspectives, not just your own.
3. Identify and examine carefully all of the ethical issues attached to the situation. Refer to your profession's code of ethics.
4. Take some time for self-reflection. Be aware of your own biases and reactions to the situation.
5. Develop several courses of action that would resolve the ethical dilemma.
6. Analyse these courses of action. Consider the short- and long-term consequences of taking such action.
7. It is a very good idea to consult other professionals in the field.
8. Choose a course of action and implement it.
9. Accept responsibility for that action and all consequences. If there are negative consequences to your action then immediately address them.
10. Examine how the ethical dilemma arose and determine how to prevent the same type of dilemma in the future.

Essentially, your responsibility as a professional when confronted with ethical issues is to evaluate who is affected, deal with your own biases or predispositions, do something about it, and then take responsibility for the action that you took. Finally, be able to rationally defend what you have done.

ETHICAL DECISION-MAKING STEPS

1. Identify the individuals and groups potentially affected by the decision.
2. Identify the ethically troubling issues, including the interests of people who will be affected by the decisions and the circumstances in which the dilemmas arose.
3. Consider how your personal biases, stresses or self-interest may influence the development of choices of action.
4. Develop alternative courses of action remembering that you do not have to do this alone. (Where feasible, include interdisciplinary team members, clients and others who may be affected by the decisions to share in the process. If the situation is difficult, consult your professional association or other trusted professionals to maintain your objectivity and increase your options for action.)
5. Analyse the likely risks and benefits of each course of action on the people likely to be affected.
6. Choose a course of action, individually or collectively, as deemed appropriate to the situation, after conscientious application of existing principles, values and standards.
7. Act, with an individual or collective commitment, to assume responsibility for the consequences of the action. (A collective commitment, as may occur within an interdisciplinary team, requires that someone be assigned the responsibility for follow-up.)
8. Establish a plan to evaluate the results of the course of action, including responsibility for correcting negative consequences, if any.
9. Evaluate the organizational systems in which the issue arose in order to identify and remedy the circumstances, which may facilitate and reward unethical practices.

Two examples of ethical decision-making models are:

- Canadian Association of Rehabilitation Professionals – http://www.carpnational.org
- Canadian Psychological Association – http://www.cpa.ca.

Two other non-psychological models of ethical decision-making can be found in Mattison (2000) and Jaeger (2001).

CODES OF ETHICS

Disability management is not yet a fully established discipline. Many DM practitioners are members of other professions such as nursing, psychology or other health professions. As a result, codes of ethics specific to DM are hard to find. However, there are two currently available. One is that of the Canadian Association of Disability Management Coordinators (CADMC) and can be found on their website at http://www.cadmc.com/code.htm

and is reproduced at the end of this chapter, with their permission, as the Appendix. Please note that this is an aspirational code and that the CADMC has no ability to enforce this code. However, it serves as a good starting point and may inform the development of other codes.

There is also the Occupational Standards for Disability Management, first promulgated by the National Institute of Disability Management and Research and accepted by the International Labour Organization.

CONCLUSION

This chapter has attempted to explain the history of ethics, how we have come to develop our understanding of what is right and wrong, and how this is reflected in professional practice. Codes of ethics and their enforcement are defining features of any profession. Disability management, perhaps because it has drawn practitioners from so many different professions, has not yet coalesced around a professional standard of practice. The time has come to do so.

APPENDIX (Part I) Canadian Association of Disability Management Coordinators Code of Ethics

Members of the CADMC are expected to adhere to the following code of ethics:

Standards of practice establish fundamental concepts and rules considered essential to promote the highest ethical standards among Disability Management Coordinators.

The standards of practice in Disability Management recognize the need to identify ethical aria [sic] professional codes of conduct as well as the need to present reasonable steps in resolving ethical dilemmas.

Ethical behaviour is a requirement of effective and competent disability management practice. Ethical and professional standards of practice dictate that the Disability Management Coordinator applies knowledge and skills in an ethical manner, recognizes that there are ethical dilemmas inherent in their professional practice and utilizes ethical decision-making to resolve ethical dilemmas. The major functions of the ethical code are to:

- protect individuals who are receiving disability management services
- provide guidance to professionals who are confronted by ethical dilemmas
- establish stakeholder and public trust and faith in the profession of disability management
- establish professional conduct between stakeholders and other professionals.

Standards of ethical practice for Disability Management Coordinators function within the following broad categories and specific rules:

1. The DMC will respect the integrity and promote and protect the welfare of individuals with whom they are working.

   - The DMC has a professional and personal responsibility and commitment to workers to implement and maintain optimal standards of disability management practice.

   - The DMC has a primary obligation to keep confidential and to safeguard information about individuals obtained in the course of disability management practice or research.

   - The DMC will ensure that the individual is aware of and understands the limits of confidentiality at the onset of disability management planning.

   - The DMC will communicate personal or confidential information to others only with the individual's written consent, or when there is a clear and immediate danger to the individual or others.

   - The DMC will discuss communication of information with the worker and will safeguard access to information, records, or other information storage means to ensure that access to information by unauthorized individuals is safeguarded.

   - The DMC shall report to the appropriate authority actions of the worker that may cause injury to self or others, after discussion with the worker that this action be taken.

   - The DMC will strive to eliminate attitudinal barriers including stereotyping and discrimination toward workers with disabilities, and will not discriminate in the provision of disability management services on the basis on disability, race, origin, religion, gender, age or sexual orientation.

2. The DMC will maintain an objective and professional standard in his/her relationship with the individuals with whom they work.

   ■ The DMC shall only provide those services that are within the scope of their competencies considering the level of education, experience and training and shall communicate the limitations imposed by the extent of their skills and knowledge in a professional area.

   ■ The DMC will ensure that individuals with whom they work understand the legal limitations and the extent and range of services that may be offered or provided in order to promote realistic expectations and open communication.

   ■ The DMC will terminate disability case management activity when the individual can no longer benefit from these services.

   ■ The DMC must clearly self-define the nature of duties, responsibilities and loyalties in order to minimize conflict of interest among management, labour, supervisors, health care providers and other stakeholders.

   ■ The DMC will refer workers or individuals with whom they may work who may compromise an objective relationship to other professionals.

3. The DMC will assist workers who are injured or disabled in developing individualized disability management or return-to-work plans that are consistent with the individual's ability and that have a reasonable probability of success.

   ■ The DMC will develop return-to-work plans and employment positions that are consistent with the abilities, limitations, interests, skills, experience and training of their worker that promote the interests of the worker; and that are consistent with the productivity and business needs of the employer.

   ■ The DMC will collaborate with the worker, physician and employer to ensure that realistic goals are set for the worker.

   ■ The DMC will advocate and promote the individual's involvement and full participation in developing return-to-work plans.

   ■ The DMC shall ensure that the worker is fully informed about all reasonable options and services available in the delivery or disability management services.

   ■ The DMC will inform workers and their families where appropriate of the benefits, implications and effects of the benefits and employment status (if any) by participation in disability management activities.

4. The DMC is obligated to promote and protect the employability of the worker by identifying and communicating the individual's abilities and limitations and by developing plans that are consistent with the interests of the worker and employer.

   ■ The DMC will develop return-to-work plans that are consistent with worker qualifications and ability to perform at work demand levels in a safe workplace.

   ■ The DMC will utilize every resource reasonably available to ensure that identified needs of workers are met including referral to other professionals or providers that may provide services or resources to maximize effective service delivery.

- The DMC shall verify the worker's needs and resources or supports needed, by using direct and valid assessments or evaluation procedures to confirm the reasonableness of the plan.

- The DMC will communicate with the employer and workplace only that information that ensures suitability to perform essential work. Informed consent will be acquired for release of any confidential information.

- The DMC will consider the safety and welfare of the worker, fellow workers and the workplace in developing return-to-work plans or in placing the worker on a job.

5. The DMC will provide disability management services within the framework of a professional relationship.

- The DMC will clarify professional relationships with workers and other stakeholders and will avoid dual relationships that could impair professional judgment or risk exploitation.

- The DMC shall cooperate with members of other professions when appropriate and shall actively participate in a collaborative team process when the worker's needs require such involvement.

- The DMC will ensure that there is a clear and mutual understanding of the disability management plans on the part of the worker and all participants in the plan, and that all plans are developed with mutual understanding and appropriate participation.

- The DMC will ensure that participants involved in the disability management plan are capable of providing maximum effective services and will ensure that the level of service expectation and outcomes is mutually understood.

6. The DMC will promote the involvement and contribution of all professionals, programs, agencies and referral sources involved with the worker who is injured or disabled to promote and provide procedures and programs that will ensure maximum benefit of services for the worker.

- The DMC shall observe ethical standards and professional conduct in interactions with other professionals involved with the worker and workplace.

- The DMC shall encourage practice, observation and promotion of ethical standards that promote the development of the disability management profession.

- The DMC will not disparage or demean other professionals, agencies or organizations or the quality of their involvement in disability management to the worker or others with whom they work.

7. The DMC is obligated to maintain his or her skills, competencies and professional development at a level to ensure that the individuals with whom he or she works benefits from the highest quality of service.

- The DMC will accurately identify the services in which the DMC is competent and qualified to perform.

- The DMC will continuously strive to maintain knowledge, develop skills and be aware of developments, resources and disability management practices that are essential to providing the highest quality of services to workers.

- The DMC will encourage individuals under their supervision to engage in activities that further the individual's professional development.

8. The DMC will promote and participate in efforts to expand the knowledge and resources needed to increase the effectiveness of services and programs for workers who are injured or disabled.

   - The DMC will institute and participate in procedures on an ongoing basis to evaluate, promote and enhance the quality of disability management services delivered in the workplace.

9. The DMC will obey all laws and regulations and will avoid activity or conduct that will cause unjust harm to others.

   - The DMC will restrict the communication of information to what is necessary and relevant with respect to the individual's right to privacy.

   - The DMC, in the performance of professional activity, shall not participate in fraudulent, deceitful, dishonest or misrepresentative actions of any kind or any form of conduct that adversely reflects on the field of disability management.

   - The DMC will not abuse the relationship with a worker to promote personal or financial gain, or financial gain for an employer.

   - The DMC shall not allow personal benefit or financial gain to interfere with professional conduct, judgment or actions.

   - The DMC shall be subjected to disciplinary actions for violations of laws, regulations, statutes or professional codes that implicate the individual's professional conduct in the future.

   - The DMC will refuse to participate in employment or business practices that conflict with moral, ethical or legal standards regarding the employer including practices that result in illegal or implied discrimination in any employment practices.

10. The DMC will demonstrate ethical and moral conduct in his or her profession.

    - The DMC will be truthful and accurate in all public statements and promotions concerning the services, programs, products and profession related to disability management.

    - The DMC shall not recommend or provide professional support for individuals who engage in professional practice that violates ethical and professional codes of practice.

    - The DMC shall inform the worker or professional committee (upon request) of ethical violations upon investigation.

APPENDIX (Part II) Code of Professional Conduct
Certification of Disability Management Specialists Commission (CDMSC)
http://www.cdms.org/ethics.htm

PREAMBLE

Throughout this document and for the purposes of this document, "client" is used to refer to the individual for whom a CDMS certificant provides services; likewise, "payor" is used to refer to the CDMS certificant's customer.

CDMS certificants recognize that their actions or inactions can either aid or hinder clients in achieving their objectives, and they accept this responsibility as part of their professional obligation. CDMS certificants may be called upon to provide a variety of services and they are obligated to do so in a manner that is consistent with their education, formal training, and work experience. In providing services, CDMS certificants must demonstrate their adherence to certain standards. The CDMSC Code of Professional Conduct has been designed to achieve these goals.

The basic objective of the Code is to protect the public interest. Accordingly the Code consists of two kinds of standards: Principles and Rules of Professional Conduct (RPCs).

The Principles are fundamental assumptions to guide professional conduct. They are advisory in nature.

The Rules of Professional Conduct prescribe the level of professional conduct required of every certificant. These Rules shall apply to all modes of communication including, but not limited to, written, oral, electronic, telephonic and Internet communications.

Compliance with this level of conduct is mandatory and will be enforced through the CDMSC Procedures for Processing Complaints.

PRINCIPLES

Principle 1: Certificants shall endeavor to place the public interest above their own at all times.

Principle 2: Certificants shall respect the integrity and protect the welfare of those persons or groups with whom they are working.

Principle 3: Certificants shall always maintain objectivity in their relationships with clients.

Principle 4: Certificants shall act with integrity in dealing with other professionals so as to facilitate their contributions with respect to achieving maximum benefits for the client.

Principle 5: Certificants shall keep their technical competency at a level which ensures their clients will receive the benefit of the highest quality of service the profession can offer.

Principle 6: Certificants shall honor the integrity and respect the limitations placed on the use of the CDMS designation.

Principle 7: Certificants shall obey all laws and regulations, avoiding any conduct or activity that could harm others.

Principle 8: Certificants shall help maintain the integrity of the Code of Professional Conduct.

RULES OF PROFESSIONAL CONDUCT

RPC 1 – Representation of Practice

Certificants shall practice only within the boundaries of their competence, based on their education, training, appropriate professional experience, and other professional credentials. They shall not misrepresent their role or competence to clients. They shall not attribute the possession of the certification designation to a depth of knowledge, skills, and professional capabilities greater than those demonstrated by achievement of certification.

RPC 2 – Competence

Certificants shall not:

a. handle or neglect a case in such a manner that the certificant's conduct constitutes gross negligence (which for the purposes of this rule shall mean willful, wanton or reckless disregard of the certificant's obligations and responsibilities).

b. exhibit a pattern of negligence or neglect in the handling of the certificant's obligations or responsibilities.

RPC 3 – Representation of Qualifications

Certificants shall neither claim nor imply professional qualifications which exceed those possessed and shall take all necessary steps to correct any misrepresentation of these qualifications. It is expected that a certificant who becomes aware of a misstatement of credentials will inform the CDMSC.

RPC 4 – Legal and Benefit System Requirements

Certificants shall work in accordance with applicable state and federal laws and the unique requirements of the various reimbursement systems involved.

RPC 5 – Testimony

Certificants, when providing testimony in a judicial or non-judicial forum, shall be impartial and limit testimony to their specific fields of expertise.

RPC 6 – Dual Relationships

Certificants who provide services at the request of a third-party payor shall disclose the nature of their dual relationship by describing their role and responsibilities to each party involved in the dual relationship. Dual relationships, other than payor/client, include, but are not limited to, certificants working with clients who are the certificant's employer, employee, friend, relative, and/or research subject, and must also be disclosed.

RPC 7 – Description of Services

Certificants shall explain services to be provided to the extent reasonably necessary to permit the client to make informed decisions, understand the purpose, techniques, rules, procedures, expected outcomes, billing arrangements, and limitations of the services rendered and identify to whom and for what purpose the results of the services will be communicated.

RPC 8 – Objectivity

Certificants shall maintain objectivity in their professional relationships and shall not impose their values on their clients.

RPC 9 – Business Relationships with Clients

Certificants shall not enter into a commercial enterprise or business relationship with any client within one year subsequent to file closure.

RPC 10 – Confidentiality: Legal Compliance

Certificants shall be knowledgeable about and act in accordance with federal, state, and local laws and procedures related to the scope of their practices regarding client consent, confidentiality, and the release of information.

RPC 11 – Confidentiality: Disclosure

Certificants shall inform the client, at the outset of the certificant–client relationship, that any information obtained through the relationship may be disclosed to third parties. Disclosure of information shall be limited to what is necessary and relevant, except that the certificant must reveal information to appropriate authorities, as soon as and to the extent that the certificant reasonably believes necessary, to prevent the client from: a) committing acts likely to result in bodily harm or imminent danger to the client or others; and b) committing criminal, illegal, or fraudulent acts.

RPC 12 – Confidentiality: Client Identity

Certificants shall omit the identity of the client when using data for training, research, publication, and/or marketing unless a written release is obtained from the client.

RPC 13 – Confidentiality: Records

Certificants shall maintain client records, whether written, taped, computerized, or stored in any other medium, in a manner designed to insure confidentiality.

RPC 14 – Reports

Certificants shall be accurate, honest, and unbiased in reporting the results of their professional activities to appropriate third parties.

RPC 15 – Electronic Recording

Certificants shall not surreptitiously record communications with clients.

RPC 16 – Records: Maintenance

Certificants shall maintain records necessary for rendering professional services to their clients and as required by applicable laws and/or regulations.

RPC 17 – Records: Storage and Disposal

Certificants shall maintain records after the file has been closed for the number of years consistent with jurisdictional requirements or for a longer period during which maintenance of such records is necessary or helpful to provide reasonably anticipated future services to the client. After that time, records shall be destroyed in a manner assuring preservation of confidentiality.

RPC 18 – Use of CDMS Designation

The designation of Certified Disability Management Specialist and the initials "CDMS" are personal in nature and may only be used by a currently certified individual. The certificant shall not utilize the designation or initials as part of a company, partnership, or corporate name, trademark, or logo.

RPC 19 – Research: Legal Compliance

Certificants shall plan, design, conduct, and report research in a manner consistent with ethical principles and federal and state laws and regulations, including those governing research with human subjects.

RPC 20 – Research: Subject Confidentiality

Certificants who make original data available, report research results, or contribute to research in any other way shall omit the identity of the subjects unless an appropriate authorization has been obtained.

RPC 21 – Misconduct

Certificants shall not commit professional misconduct. It is professional misconduct if the certificant:

a) violates or attempts to violate the Code of Professional Conduct, knowingly assists or induces another to do so, or does so through the acts of another;

b) commits a criminal act that reflects adversely on the certificant's honesty or trustworthiness;

c) engages in conduct involving dishonesty, fraud, deceit, or misrepresentation;

d) engages in conduct involving discrimination against a client because of race, color, religion, age, gender, sexual orientation, national origin, marital status, or disability;

e) engages in sexually intimate behavior with a client; or

f) accepts as a client an individual with whom the certificant has been sexually intimate.

RPC 22 – Conflict of Interest

Certificants shall fully disclose an actual or potential conflict of interest to all affected parties. If, after full disclosure, an objection is made by any affected party, the certificant shall withdraw from further participation in the case.

RPC 23 – Termination of Services

Certificants shall recommend the termination of case activity when the certificant reasonably believes that the client is no longer benefiting or when services are no longer required.

RPC 24 – Fees

Certificants shall advise the payor of their fee structure in advance of the rendering of any services and shall also furnish, upon request, detailed, accurate time and expense records.

RPC 25 – Advertising

Certificants who describe/advertise services shall do so in a manner that accurately informs the public of the services, expertise, and techniques being offered. Descriptions/advertisements by a certificant shall not contain false, inaccurate, misleading, out-of-context, or otherwise deceptive material or statements. If statements from former clients are to be used, the certificant shall have a written, signed, and dated release from the former clients. All advertising shall be factually accurate and shall not contain exaggerated claims as to costs and/or results.

RPC 26 – Solicitation

Certificants shall neither solicit nor accept commissions, rebates, or any form of remuneration for the referral of clients for professional services.

RPC 27 – Reporting Misconduct

Certificants possessing personal knowledge concerning a violation or any potential violation of the CDMSC Code of Professional Conduct by a certificant shall report such information to the CDMSC.

RPC 28 – Compliance with Proceedings

Certificants shall assist in the process of enforcing the CDMSC Code of Professional Conduct by cooperating with investigations, participating in proceedings, and complying with the directives of the Committee for Professional Conduct.

RPC 29 – Frivolous Complaints

Certificants shall not initiate, participate in, or encourage the filing of complaints that are malicious, unwarranted, or without a basis in fact.

REFERENCES

Botes A 2000 A comparison between the ethics of justice and the ethics of care. Journal of Advanced Nursing 32(5):1071–1075

Hermeren G 1999 Setting priorities versus managing closures: what is ethically the most sound way of handling changes in the health care system? Acta Onocologica 38(1):33–40

Huycke L, All A C 2000 Quality in health care and ethical principles. Journal of Advanced Nursing 32(3):562–571

Jaeger S M 2001 Teaching health care ethics: the importance of moral sensitivity for moral reasoning. Nursing Philosophy 2:131–142

Kant I 1949 On a supposed right to lie from altruistic motives. In: Kant I, Critique of Practical Reason and Other Writings in Moral Philosophy (White B L, trans.). University of Chicago Press, Chicago

Kant I 1959 Foundations of the Metaphysics of Morals (White B L, trans.). Bobbs-Merrill, Indianapolis

Noziak R 1974 Anarchy State and Utopia. Basic Books, New York

Mattison M 2000 Ethical decision-making: the person in the process. Social Work 45(3):201–212

Chapter 16

Future trends in disability management

Disability management (DM) is an evolving field. As such it is constantly being confronted with new issues. Originally conceived as an attempt to assist workers with worksite injures to return to work (RTW), DM has proven to be extremely successful and has grown to include all aspects of disability, and is now practised throughout the world. In an attempt to get a sense of what the future holds for DM we asked several people active in DM, in various ways and in varied locations, to give us their views of new and emerging trends in DM. What follows are their contributions.

NICHOLAS BUYS
Associate Professor and Head of the School of Human Services at Griffith University, Meadowbrook, Queensland, Australia

FUTURE OF DISABILITY MANAGEMENT IN AUSTRALIA

Disability management has been viewed as something of a panacea for reducing escalating workers' compensation and disability costs in Australia. Over the last two decades both Commonwealth and State Governments have focused on expanding and improving services that prevent injuries, retain injured employees at the workplace and assist people with disabilities to obtain work. Much of this focus has been on legislative and regulatory changes to encourage safer workplaces, improve injury management and case-management practices, and reduce disincentives to obtain work. However, the results of these efforts have been patchy. For example, although the number of workers' compensation claims has decreased between 1998–1999 and 2002–2003 the average numbers of days of paid compensation and the costs of claims and premiums have risen. Although there have been declines in many injury categories, there have been increases in the incidence of occupational overuse syndrome, stress and disease claims. Evidence suggests that the number of workplace injuries and diseases is much higher than the number eligible for workers' compensation, with the annual economic cost of workplace injuries estimated to be over Aus\$30 billion (Productivity Commission 2004).

The future of DM in Australia is about addressing the above issues, and, with this in mind, the following strategies are suggested. Governments and employers need to implement comprehensive disability management (CDM) programmes rather than adopt a piecemeal approach. Although there are examples of excellent DM programmes in Australia (Westmorland & Buys 2002), employer-based prevention, health promotion and occupational rehabilitation services are usually not well integrated to prevent and manage injury and illness. Furthermore, there needs to be more emphasis on employer–labour collaboration to promote DM. A recent review of workers' compensation arrangements in Australia recognized the importance of a cooperative approach in recommending that 'return to work programs be developed and implemented by a committed partnership of the employer, employee and treating doctor . . .' (Productivity Commission 2004: 213). This approach strengthens 'occupational bonds' between management and workers, and contributes to higher RTW rates and more durable RTW outcomes.

Unfortunately, common law access in some Australian state workers' compensation schemes and employers' unwillingness to guarantee employment security for injured workers (Purse 2002) has created, in some instances, an adversarial atmosphere between management and labour has hindered the development of consensus-based DM programmes. Abolition of common-law access combined with increased employer responsibility for supporting rehabilitation of injured workers is critical to an effective injury management programme (Productivity Commission 2004).

Employers need more support and financial incentives to implement DM programmes. Many Australian state workers' compensation systems have bonus and penalty systems in place. Employers who reduce claims incidence and costs can obtain a reduction in their premiums, while poor-performing employers are penalized by an increase in their premiums. Although these are positive incentives, additional measures are needed that reward employers for implementing high-quality, CDM programmes. This type of scheme, an example of which is being piloted in British Columbia, Canada, provides premium discounts for those provincial employers who meet specific DM standards (Workers' Compensation Board of British Columbia 2004).

Development of more effective DM strategies is required to meet costly, high-incidence injury areas such as stress conditions. Much of the focus of DM to date has been on the prevention and management of physical injuries and disease. However, the management of stress-related injuries will require different approaches by employers. Given that occupational wellbeing is linked to high morale and work–life balance, DM interventions for stress need to focus on creating healthy organizations for people to work in as well as 'treat' the individual. Indeed, employers will need to incorporate broad-based organizational change strategies as part of their DM programmes to develop positive workplace cultures that minimize the incidence of stress conditions.

The success of DM in the future will rely on its ability to accommodate the needs of people with chronic conditions. Over the last 25 years there has been an increased prevalence in chronic conditions among Australians, largely as a result of improvements in medical knowledge and diagnosis, and reduced mortality rates (Wen 2004). With the shrinking pool of available labour over the next two decades employers will need to retain workers with chronic conditions. Disability management programmes will need to focus organizational responses on areas such as suitable job accommodations and flexible work hours, ensuring that workers with such conditions are able to continue to contribute productively to the workplace.

Finally, the future of DM will depend on its ability to rigorously demonstrate effective outcomes for injured workers and organizations. This will require research approaches that withstand public scrutiny. To date, research in this area has been hampered by a number of problems including multiple definitions of DM, lack of an explicit theory base and conceptual framework, lack of rigour in research design and few appropriate measurement instruments. Significant work is needed to address these issues.

REFERENCES

Productivity Commission 2004 National Workers' Compensation and Occupational Health and Safety Frameworks, Report No. 27. Australian Government, Canberra

Purse K 2002 Workers compensation-based employment security for injured workers: a review of legislation and enforcement. Journal of Occupational Health and Safety – Australia and New Zealand 18(1):61–66

Wen X 2004 Trends in the prevalence of disability and chronic conditions among the older population: implications for survey design and measurement of disability. Australasian Journal on Ageing 23(1):3–6

Westmorland M, Buys N 2002 Disability management in a sample of Australian self-insured companies. Disability and Rehabilitation 24(14):746–754

Workers' Compensation Board of British Columbia 2004 WCB introduces incentives to assist successful return to work (press release, 20 January)

STEFAN KESSLER
Co-owner and Director of Rehafirst AG/Zürich
He is responsible for case management projects at the workplace and for individual case management especially after accidents.

HANS SCHMIDT
Co-owner of Rehafirst AG/Zürich
He is an economist and claimant's lawyer. As a lawyer he tries to reintegrate his client with the help of a team of case managers. At the same time he tries to convince insurance companies to change their claims management from 'deny and defend' to 'accept and assist'.

DISABILITY MANAGEMENT IN SWITZERLAND – FUTURE PROSPECTS

Case management as a method of DM is more and more accepted and disseminated in Switzerland. However, if its main aim is to avoid disability there is a long way to go. In future the chances are based on the one hand in a change of mentality of insurance companies' attitudes and on the other hand on profoundly elaborated business management concepts of enterprises and institutions.

Mainly, accident insurers have nowadays recognized that they can no longer rely on the ailing – and in many cases helpless – national disability insurance company, which has by law the monopoly on reintegration and RTW programmes. If they pay no respect to this fact, they and their client often end up as losers. Winners are the representatives of the medical system and the lawyers, who have managed to save their fee. With the help of case management this situation can change for the better. Therefore, in Switzerland, a change of mentality is taking place in insurance companies, especially in the accident and liability sectors. This change is based on two pillars:

- Process orientation instead of split-up competence, which means that a case manager is responsible for the whole process of reintegration.
- Early management instead of passivity, which means that the case manager starts his or her accompaniment as soon as the assessment of damage is effected, preferably 14 days after the event.

However, experts in reintegration agree that these two changes in mentality are not enough. In order to achieve a successful case management in the insurance business there are five steps to take:

1. *From deficit orientation to resource orientation* The case manager consequently activates the existing skills of the person affected instead of questioning deficits and problems.
2. *Getting away from the medical expert system towards a holistic view of the person affected* Profession and private environment are as important as the medical field.
3. *Work as a step towards rehabilitation instead of medical rehabilitation before work* A step-by-step return towards work gives better results than the endless waiting to become totally well again. This idea, at the moment, is revolutionary for the whole insurance/medical community.
4. *The parallel management of scenarios instead of waiting for reports from experts* A professional and private setting of the course must take place during the acute phase before physicians, always delayed, offer solutions based on 'deficit thinking'.
5. *Acceptance of disability* The 'hot potato' – an irreversible disability must be discussed. The question is if the client can accept being able to lead a meaningful life regardless of the disability. The medical system and insurers tend to follow the course of a 150% back-to-performance strategy. Clients are eager to follow this dangerous and blinkered mentality. When you feel strong pain one day you have to think about accepting handicaps.

We know from practice that with this change in mentality, longterm chronic cases are brought back into the light. Taking into consideration these successes, we can be optimistic that at least some insurers are capable of fulfilling this change in mentality and profit from this advantage of competition.

GREATER IMPACT – AVOIDING DISABILITY IN COMPANIES

Insurance companies are facing two handicaps. First, they can only take on cases when damages are big, which means that professional, health and social damage is already substantial. Second, the goodwill of reintegration through insurers is questioned by the person affected. Workers may think that insurers only think about cost-cutting.

Therefore, in Switzerland, new ways must be found to reach this aim. We are convinced that the greatest impact and the biggest chance of success in respect to reintegration are given when employers undertake concrete steps to avoid disability. The advantages for employers as compared to insurers are obvious:

- *Early diagnosis of health problems* On the job it soon becomes obvious if an employee is limited for health reasons. Therefore the questions of threatening disability can be asked at an earlier stage and the situation can be managed actively.
- *Intact professional life* If an employee becomes a case for a case manager, there usually exists an intact professional surrounding. The person affected is a member of a team who has a good reputation and is accepted.
- *Confidence* There often exists a situation of confidence between the employee and the supervisor, a confidence that has grown during a long time spent working together. This confidence is indispensable in order to achieve successful reintegration.

How, in practice, can companies profit from these advantages and why should they care?

A successful translation into practice asks for clear solutions in business management. These solutions have to be adapted individually in each company, in its culture, economic conditions and marketing solutions, e.g. ready-made solutions do not exist. But there are several common values that have to be considered in such a concept:

- Intersection to presence management, e.g. signalling possible problem cases at an early stage.
- Integration of disability avoidance into a reporting system, e.g. codes and quality factors by which the effectiveness of company case management can be measured, such as a balanced score-card.
- Organizational classification of case manager: internal or external depending on partnership with another company.
- Distribution of the costs of case management among all those who are profiting from the new system, e.g. in Switzerland this also involves the benefit plan system.

The last point at least partially answers the second point – a company should tend to care actively about avoiding in-house disability as it helps to cut direct and indirect costs, e.g. insurance premiums, and efforts to replace an employee and the costs of absence management. Today, when case management in companies may still sound somewhat exotic, the effort of the reintegration of an employee can create a positive impression on the staff: 'We care for you!'. It certainly adds credibility and image to a company.

Some companies and organizations are already starting pilot projects of case management. The coming years will show if case management in companies can win a position in economic reality. This means cutting costs and offering employees a better life.

A MAJOR PUBLIC SECTOR EMPLOYER

FUTURE TRENDS IN DISABILITY MANAGEMENT

For many years we have managed what is measured with respect to lost-time injuries and severity impacting safety performance. Too often DM programmes are a reaction to these measures. A shift towards an integrated approach to DM, where all disease or injuries are managed consistently, is reality today.

DOWNSIZING AND THE AGEING WORKFORCE

As a publicly owned company rapid change is commonplace. Downsizing and early retirement schemes made the bottom line seem attractive but have reduced the number of experienced and skilled staff. The remaining employees often perform work of more than one person while engaging in overtime. The ageing workforce will face the reality of illness, disease, stress and injury associated with age and a very stressful work environment.

The trend towards an ageing workforce will result in an increase in occupational and non-occupational injury, disease and illness. The Workplace Safety and Insurance reporting obligations are legislated. We have developed a programme to facilitate the reporting of injuries including claims management and early and safe RTW programmes. Although the legislated segment of our absences are managed, the number of injuries and permanent disabilities continues to rise.

LEGISLATION AND COLLECTIVE AGREEMENTS

On the non-occupational side, collective agreements determine the extent of benefits paid. Often these plans can be generous. Universal DM programmes are designed to manage all injuries or disease with a consistent model. Legislation and collective agreements set the bar but it is incumbent that we manage these absences as cost-effectively as possible. This will be accomplished by teamwork, hiring external providers when required and using in-house resources to the fullest.

Further reductions in disability costs, both human and financial, will require teamwork and, potentially, changes to collective agreements. In order to stay competitive with an ageing, injured and ill workforce, collective bargaining will need to address benefit packages and ensure that they are supportive of integrated DM efforts. It is important that illness and injury management continue. Additionally, the extent of benefit may need to be reduced to give workers an incentive to RTW. As the number of claimants continues to increase, new innovative approaches will be required to improve health and reduce disability. Lobbying governments who set the legislation along with changes to the insurance acts should continue. Employers working together empowered in lobby groups can help effect changes with legislation that might improve the laws, facilitate better service and reduce costs.

POST-OFFER EMPLOYMENT SCREENING

Post-offer employment screening will become an important function to determine the fitness level of new employees. The first step is to identify capabilities to determine the ability to perform work then ensure that appropriate duties are assigned. If an injury occurs, a baseline has already been established. Recovery must be closely monitored to pre-injury levels and cost relief sought when appropriate.

DISABILITY MANAGEMENT TEAMS

The future of DM will require skilled and educated RTW coordinators in teams managing cases within the entitlement framework. A full range of DM services for occupational and non-occupational illness and injury is required using all the elements of a CDM programme.

WELLNESS

Wellness initiatives, with real support from management, including an understanding that investing up front is critical, can reduce the costs of illness and absence. Early detection of illness and disease through proactive wellness programmes is required. So is gathering accurate data from the DM programme to stay ahead of any new trends. For companies that do not support these initiatives the disability costs will continue to escalate.

CONCLUSION

All the above elements require hard work and support but are always cost-effective in the long run. Companies with vision and concern for their most valuable resource can do much to keep costs down while providing a safer, healthier and more accommodating workplace. An effective DM programme makes good business sense.

JEFF CURTIS
Director of Human Resources at Manitoba Telecom Services
*Jeff is a member of the senior HR team, playing a lead role in the delivery of human resources or 'people'
management for the MTS family of companies. His current responsibilities include strategic and tactical HR planning,
HR performance measurement, wellness, environment and DM, HRIS/HRIM, training and development, and employee
and family assistance programmes.*

EMERGING COMPETENCIES FOR DISABILITY MANAGEMENT PROFESSIONALS

What they didn't teach you in school

As DM professionals, we find ourselves working in a global, highly competitive and ever-changing business environment. Flowing from this, we are faced with new and emerging processes, methods, tools and techniques as well as increased requirements and expectations. The result is that we are continuously challenged to maintain the skills, knowledge and abilities necessary to excel within our profession and continue to be seen as leaders in organizational health and DM. Through this book, Drs Harder and Scott have done much to help us stay on top of our game.

Today, companies keep a constant and keen eye on how workplace programmes or initiatives impact on the bottom line and contribute to overall business goals. This includes DM. Recognizing this, some DM professionals have succeeded in taking DM to the next level by demonstrating how it can be included in corporate business plans and how it can positively influence a company's bottom line. Such an approach or model is presented in Chapter 4 (Fig. 4.5).

A history of helping

The vast majority of DM professionals have long enjoyed a respected tradition of preventing and minimizing illness and injury through occupational health interventions. Through education and experience, DM professionals come equipped to develop and implement programmes aimed at promoting and maintaining the health and safety of millions of employees in countless Canadian workplaces.

Disability management professionals have long recognized the need to effectively manage disability arising from occupational and non-occupational illness and injury, and have developed or operated under various case-management models. Moving away from more traditional models, we have all witnessed the growth of *workplace-based* efforts intended to assist workers with disabilities to return to work following the onset of illness or injury.

As a group, DM professionals are acutely aware of the alarming human and financial costs that result from disability. As a result, many DM professionals have committed themselves to minimizing the occurrence and outcome of disability through workplace-based efforts. *However, there is considerable uncertainty about whether educational programmes have adequately prepared DM professionals to succeed in a business-orientated, corporate world that measures everything.*

Emerging requirements

Let's assume that the vast majority of active DM professionals possess the requisite skills required for managing individual cases of disability. As a core competency, these professionals possess the ability to assess and determine available options, weigh options, and develop, implement and evaluate DM plans on an individual and aggregate basis.

Emerging business requirements mean that DM professionals need to develop additional competency – i.e. a cluster of knowledge, skills, abilities and aptitudes – if they want to continue playing a leading role in developing and delivering DM programmes in today's business world.

Emerging competency requirements associated with workplace-based DM include:

- organizational behaviour and development including communication strategies and tactics, employee relations, leadership development, process improvement, performance management and measurement, and strategic business planning
- programme and policy development, implementation and evaluation consistent with business goals
- business acumen including business case development, establishing return on investment (ROI) incorporating productivity and cost–benefit analysis, developing and delivering business communications, and engaging executive or senior management.

What do disability management professionals need to know today?

The rapidly growing popularity of workplace-based DM has seen people from various professional disciplines and educational backgrounds step forward as 'disability managers'.

Notwithstanding the base academic preparation received by many of these individuals, it is believed that it is not uncommon for DM professionals to find that their academic preparation did not fully prepare them for the responsibilities assumed and the performance expectations attached to managing disability in corporate business environments. This can leave DM professionals feeling frustrated, misunderstood or not respected by the business people with whom they interact.

What do DM professionals need to know to avoid such a dilemma? First and foremost, they need to be fully conversant in how today's businesses operate, the challenges that companies face in today's ever-changing business world and how DM fits into this equation. Specifically, DM professionals need to demonstrate a clear understanding of, be able to speak to, and address issues such as the following:

- the business process for preparing strategic plans and business plans including HR or 'people' management
- how DM is aligned with these business plans
- corporate requirements to make business decisions by considering business cases, ROI, cost–benefit analysis, and how each and every proposed initiative must support business objectives

- how DM is based on a solid business case including ROI, cost–benefit analysis and is one component of effective people management
- the need for today's companies to develop supervisory managers who are skilled leaders of people in addition to being technically proficient in order to achieve business objectives
- how DM is one component of a leader's responsibility to demonstrate a commitment to employees, including ensuring their welfare and wellbeing
- the need for companies to engage and satisfy employees in order to achieve business objectives
- how DM is one component in engaging employees, increasing productivity and achieving bottom-line revenue and profit targets
- the common business practice of using standard business methods and criteria to request and evaluate programme proposals from internal and external resources
- how DM proposals can be articulated through content and format that resonates with decision-makers in business
- the reality that today's companies expect internal and external service providers to be responsive, understand the workplace and culture, and be able to communicate and work effectively with employees at all levels
- how DM needs to be developed and delivered using the same business acumen and 'savvy' employed by internal or external consultants charged with addressing any business issue
- corporate Canada's increasing use of sophisticated and rigorous systems to track baselines, service delivery, costs, and outcomes for all business processes
- how DM is no different than any other business process, which must demonstrate its value through commonly accepted evaluation methods.

These are just some of the emerging competency requirement considerations for DM professionals if they want to continue to be successful in gaining and sustaining commitment to effective DM in Canada's workplaces.

WHY SHOULD WE CARE ABOUT THESE NEW REQUIREMENTS?

Aside from the inherent desire to continuously build on their capabilities in order to meet the needs of workers with disabilities, DM professionals will lose credibility and the ability to promote and implement DM if they cannot continue to effectively navigate business environments. As a group of professionals, we must be sensitive to 'business' and be articulate in business acumen. Without this, it will be the workers with disabilities and Canada's economy that will be the losers.

JANE VOS
Vice-President of Operations for Organizational Solutions

She has been participating in the DM practice area for over 15 years, assisting multiple employers in her current DM consulting role.

Disability management, although still a young profession, has made many significant inroads to improve outcomes for individuals and companies that are plagued with disabilities and disability-related issues. Intense interventions in prevention, claim initiation, claim/care management, RTW and rehabilitation are the primary foundations that are taking significant root in the field of DM.

Prevention requires employers to look at management practices and ensure they are supporting a healthy workplace. Current workplace research indicates the one most important variable in absence or RTW is relationships in the workplace. Identification of workplace relationship conflicts is critical at the onset of claim management as this will guide the management and control of the claim. Differentiating between labour relations issues and true disability issues has proven to have significant impact on disability claim entitlement and the duration of absence should a disability occur.

Clearly, the more detail that is gathered on claim initiation, the more likely sound, information-based claim decisions will be made.

Claims management has been taken to a higher and leading-edge level at Organizational Solutions where the model in managing disability claims is handled from a care management perspective instead of the traditional 'case or claim' management approach.

This model moves away from 'paper file management' to a 'high-touch personal' approach with immediate claim intervention at the claim initiation phase.

This care management innovation is vital in today's disability environment as it provides the disability care manager with a holistic approach to disease management and RTW.

Many evidence-based best practices are evolving for the treatment of specific conditions in disease management. The care management model provides a valuable and informative venue in raising employees' and physicians' levels of awareness of these best practices.

Changes to workers' compensation legislation (about 10 years ago) have mandated that employees and employers participate together in RTW planning. This process has been highly successful on the occupational side. To positively impact the outcomes of all disabilities, the above strategies need to be universally streamlined to also include non-occupational claims.

While assisting and working closely with Dr Scott over recent years, I have observed the care management model significantly impacting on DM in North America. The incorporation of this unique care management model has resulted in a tremendous economical impact for major corporations throughout Canada and the USA, taking these organizations to world-class status in disability claims management.

DR JUR. FRIEDRICH MEHRHOFF
HVBG (German Federation of Institutions – for statutory accident insurance and prevention)

Germany looks back at over a century of tradition in social security. In this context the name Bismarck was known throughout the world. One of the key elements of this tradition is the responsibility of social partners within the social insurance carriers. They are neither run by the state nor by profit-orientated private insurers.

The workers' compensation boards in Germany, covering the risk of accidents at work or of occupational diseases, have been focusing on case-management strategies for decades. Their representatives, i.e. the employers' and employees' delegates, establish rules in prevention and rehabilitation in order to contribute to the workforce of the German population.

The German statutory accident insurers employ about 3000 people who advise worksites in matters of safety and in the challenges of returning to work after an injury or disease related to work. Together with service providers they set quality standards in DM. The international exchange provides the chance to find out if an organization or system is really as good as its representatives think.

What needs to be done to take DM to the next level of success and what can Germany contribute to this process?

- The public employers, as well as social insurers, have to be a shining example to private companies. They should introduce DM programmes first.
- Economics can help convince employers to accept an efficient DM programme. Financial thinking and social concerns are not mutually exclusive.
- Disability management must be consensus-based to avoid restrictions within an organization. Employees (and unions) must be convinced that DM provides longterm outcomes instead of just absence management.
- The goal of DM has to be an 'ability' management which concentrates on what disabled persons can achieve, because looking only at what they cannot do creates unnecessary barriers.
- Physicians should be involved in DM activities. Their credibility with the disabled community and with occupational health doctors increases the likelihood of a more successful RTW.
- Links to prevention strategies in the organization will have a synergetic effect on DM activities; both elements are two sides of the same coin.
- Disability management can only be successful if government, social partners, insurers, service providers and researchers work together. Legal principles have to be put into practice by 'round tables' within companies.
- Education is one milestone toward the future in DM. Programmes with bachelors' and masters' degrees allow for the exchange of students and experiences all over the world.

- Employers should not delegate their responsibility of DM to disability managers. In order to do so they need financial incentives. Therefore an audit can measure their efforts and successes and lead to lower insurance premiums.
- International organizations have to be involved in DM standards so that together with the WHO, ILO, RI or ISSA the next steps can be made and will be accepted around the world.

The Third International Forum on DM in Australia in 2006 and the fourth in Germany in 2008 will provide the platform for discussing these and other priorities. Let's focus not only on the big organizations but also implement DM in small and medium-sized companies. It is important to look for strategic partners in DM worldwide. The German workers' compensation boards feel responsible and open for DM exchange.

LINDA NKEMDRIM
Occupational Health Services Manager, Canadian Pacific Railway

FUTURE OF DISABILITY MANAGEMENT

When asked for my opinion on the future of disability management, my thoughts immediately turn to my personal desires, rather than what I think is likely to happen. Therefore, my opinion on the future of disability management is two-fold, from personal and professional perspectives.

Looking at disability management objectively and professionally, I think the future looks good. Why? More and more workplaces will be forced to implement some form of disability management programme, because of a number of factors. Economic factors such as the high costs of disability benefits and increased competition for the current and predicted skill and labour shortages are motivating employers into action. Employers are forced to seek non-traditional means of addressing these economic factors because the traditional solutions are no longer possible or effective. Employers are beginning to realize that it is cost-effective to accommodate their own employees and to expand their human resource strategy to include roles for minority groups such as individuals with disability.

To help employers along the way, the current Canadian political, social and economic climate is pushing governments to do more for individuals with disability through investment in healthcare, social and training programmes, as well as better enforcement of legislation.

Introduction of disability courses as well as certificate and degree programmes at the post-secondary level will result in an increase in the number of qualified disability management professionals and increased awareness of the discipline. The National Institute of Disability Management & Research's (NIDMAR) certification programme is gaining recognition and acceptance among current disability management practitioners. These developments offer better assurance to employers of the qualifications of the people they hire to manage disability.

Advancement in the medical field and the multidisciplinary approach to healthcare are helping individuals with disability to attain higher functional levels, while technological advancements such as assistive devices are improving their ability to participate more effectively in society.

As older workers retire from the workforce, so will a number of traditionally held views and values on the 'ways of doing business'. The younger workers are better educated, less likely to forge allegiance to one organization, less hung-up on tradition and more open to diversity. This means that working side by side with an individual with disability only requires the creativity to accommodate their disability.

Having been professionally involved in disability management for the past 16 years, my experience has ranged across the entire spectrum of disability management programmes, from makeshift to comprehensive. Throughout my journey with disability management, I often ask myself the same question. What is the perfect disability management programme? My personal opinion is that the perfect disability management programme is one that assists EVERY individual with an impairment to attain their optimum functional level and to participate in every aspect of society to the best of their abilities and desires. This means accommodation must extend beyond the workplace. In other words, disability management would be a seamless process that effectively integrates workplace programmes with those of society. Regardless of these musings, I remain optimistic that we are about to make major strides in disability management!

Subject Index